AF871167

Guillain-Barré Syndrome

From Diagnosis To Recovery

By
Joel S. Steinberg
Gareth J. Parry

16
EasyRead Large

RHYW

Copyright Page from the Original Book

Library of Congress Cataloging-in-Publication Data

Parry, Gareth J.

Guillain-Barré syndrome : from diagnosis to recovery / Gareth J. Parry, Joel S. Steinberg.

p. cm. — (American Academy of Neurology (AAN) quality of life guides)

Includes bibliographical references and index.

ISBN-13: 978-1-932603-56-9 (pbk. : alk. paper)

ISBN-10: 1-932603-56-5 (pbk. : alk. paper)

1. Guillain-Barré syndrome. I. Steinberg, Joel S. II. Title.

RC416.P37 2007

616.8'56—dc22

2006030462

Medicine is an ever-changing science undergoing continual development. Research and clinical experience are continually expanding our knowledge, in particular our knowledge of proper treatment and drug therapy. The authors, editors, and publisher have made every effort to ensure that all information in this book is in accordance with the state of knowledge at the time of production of the book.

Nevertheless, this does not imply or express any guarantee or responsibility on the part of the authors, editors, or publisher with respect to any dosage instructions and forms of application stated in the book. Every reader should examine carefully the package inserts accompanying each drug and check with a his physician or specialist whether the dosage schedules mentioned therein or the contraindications stated by the manufacturer differ from the statements made in this book. Such examination is particularly important with drugs that are either rarely used or have been newly released on the market. Every dosage schedule or every form of application used is entirely at the reader's own risk and responsibility. The editors and publisher welcome any reader to report to the publisher any discrepancies or inaccuracies noticed.

Made in the United States of America

07 08 09 10 5 4 3 2 1

This optimized ReadHowYouWant edition contains the complete, unabridged text of the original publisher's edition. Other aspects of the book may vary from the original edition.

Set in 16 pt. Verdana

TABLE OF CONTENTS

AMERICAN ACADEMY OF NEUROLOGY (AAN)

Quality of Life Guides
Lisa M. Shulman, MD
Series Editor

Alzheimer's Disease
Paul Dash, MD and Nicole Villemarette-Pittman, PhD

Amyotrophic Lateral Sclerosis
Robert G. Miller, MD, Deborah Gelinas, MD, and Patricia O'Connor, RN

Epilepsy
Ilo E. Leppik, MD

Guillain-Barré Syndrome
Gareth John Parry, MB, ChB, FRACP and Joel Steinberg, MD, PhD

Migraine and Other Headaches
William B. Young, MD and Stephen D. Silberstein, MD

Peripheral Neuropathy
Norman Latov, MD

Restless Legs Syndrome
Mark J. Buchfuhrer, MD, Wayne A. Hening, MD, PhD,

and Clete Kushida, MD, PhD

Stroke
Louis R. Caplan, MD

Understanding Pain
Harry J. Gould, III, MD, PhD

About the AAN Press Quality of Life Guides

IN THE SPIRIT OF THE DOCTOR-PATIENT PARTNERSHIP

The better-informed patient is often able to play a vital role in his or Ther own care. This is especially the case with neurologic disorders, for which effective management of disease can be promoted—indeed, *enhanced*—through patient education and involvement.

In the spirit of the partnership-in-care between physicians and patients, the American Academy of Neurology Press is pleased to produce a series of "Quality of Life" guides on an array of diseases and ailments that affect the brain and central nervous system. The series, produced in partnership with Demos Medical Publishing, answers a number of basic and important questions faced by patients and their families.

Additionally, the authors, most of whom are physicians and all of whom are experts in the areas in which they write, provide a detailed discussion of the disorder, its causes, and the course it may follow. You also find strategies for coping with the disorder and handling a number of non-medical issues.

The result: As a reader, you will be able to develop a framework for understanding the disease and become better prepared to manage the life changes associated with it.

ABOUT THE AMERICAN ACADEMY OF NEUROLOGY (AAN)

The American Academy of Neurology is the premier organization for neurologists worldwide. In addition to support of educational and scientific advances, the AAN—along with its sister organization, the AAN Foundation—is a strong advocate of public education and a leading supporter of research for breakthroughs in neurologic patient care.

More information on the activities of the AAN is available on our website, www.aan.com. For a better understanding of common disorders of the brain, as well as to learn about people living with these disorders, please turn to the AAN Foundation's website, w ww.thebrainmatters.org.

ABOUT NEUROLOGY AND NEUROLOGISTS

Neurology is the medical specialty associated with disorders of the brain and central nervous system. Neurologists are medical doctors with specialized training in the diagnosis, treatment, and management of patients suffering from neurologic disease.

Lisa M. Shulman, MD

Series Editor
AAN Press Quality of Life Guides

Foreword

Guillain-barre syndrome (GBS) is a rare disease by any standard, affecting about 2 in 100,000 people per year worldwide. Yet, it is now the most common cause of acute flaccid paralysis worldwide since the near-demise of polio. Neurologists have been fascinated by this disease of the peripheral nervous system since the two most cited papers; Landry in 1859 and later Guillain, Barré, and Strohl in 1916. Interest in GBS accelerated following the seminal paper of Asbury, Arnason, and Adams in 1969 showing that GBS was an immune-mediated disorder. Animal models were developed, and the science was off and running. Treatment of the human disease received a large boost with the trials of plasmapheresis in the 1980s which showed benefit compared to standard supportive treatment. In the 1990s, intravenous immunoglobulin was shown equivalent to plasmapheresis which is now the standard treatment in those places where it is available. While neurologists were concentrating on the acute phase of the disease and physiatrists on the early rehabilitation phase, patients were left to deal with GBS for the rest of their lives. Into that void stepped Estelle Benson, the wife of Robert who had developed GBS. Virtually single-handed, she created what is now a global patient-oriented group, the GBS/CIDP Foundation International (www.gbsfi.com . The foundation is a patient support group for individuals and their families with GBS and the related conditionchronicinflammatorydemyelinatingpolyneuropathy (CIDP). Early in that effort, she and Dr. Joel Steinberg, a physician who had GBS, realized that no book directly targeted patients with GBS and their families. In 1983 Joel wrote, *Guillain-Barré Syndrome: An Overview for the Layperson.* At about the same time, scientific information on GBS was accelerating but again, no single source was available. Then, three medical books on GBS were published at about the same time. *Guillain-Barré Syndrome* by Richard A.C. Hughes (1990), *Guillain-Barré Syndrome* by Allan Ropper, Eelco F.M. Wijdicks, and Bradley T. Truax (1991), and *Guillain-Barré Syndrome* by Gareth J. Parry (1993).

Guillain-Barré Syndrome: From Diagnosis to Recovery is a superb book and is the natural evolution of two threads—one scientifically-oriented and the other patient-oriented—woven together. There is something for everyone in this excellent book. Physicians and scientists will find up-todate chapters on diagnosis, treatment, and causation of GBS and CIDP. Occupational therapists, physical therapists, and others involved in rehabilitation will be drawn to the chapters discussing treatment in acute care and rehabilitation hospitals, and home and community. For patients and their families, there is the entire book!

The book is well organized, packed with useful and practical information, and written at a level that is approachable for all readers. The chapters are broken into sections with headings that help to direct the reader in finding information.

Guillain-Barré Syndrome: From Diagnosis to Recovery will be an important addition to the libraries of many interested readers. I am personally delighted to be associated in this small way with such a volume.

David R. Cornblath, MD
The Johns Hopkins University School of Medicine
Baltimore, MD

Preface

Gullain-Barre syndrome (GBS) is an uncommon disorder, but one whose impact is far out of proportion to its incidence. Despite a usually good prognosis, GBS is a particularly frightening and often life-altering experience for those diagnosed with the disorder. Many patients are acutely aware of the rapid loss of control of their muscular function, including vital functions such as breathing and swallowing, and frequently feel that they are dying. The experience is almost as unnerving for the families of affected individuals. During the acute phase of the illness GBS patients experience the indignity of helplessness in addition to their fear of death or permanent disability. Prolonged disability is common and some permanent residual effects are becoming increasingly recognized. It has been our experience in meeting patients at support groups, that individuals who have been affected by GBS have a great desire for a better understanding of the disorder, even years after the acute experience.

Chronic inflammatory demyelinating polyneuropathy (CIDP) in many ways is similar to GBS from the physicians' perspective, but is perceived quite differently by patients. Most people and many non-neurological physicians have never heard of CIDP. Many cases go undiagnosed and in other cases the diagnosis is delayed so that treatment is ineffective. It is not a dramatic illness; weakness usually evolves over months, not days, and it may be years before the true nature of the disorder is recognized and appropriate treatment instituted. This delay in treatment may have unfortunate consequences since delayed treatment may be ineffective treatment. CIDP is a life-long disease and, therefore, has a major impact on the quality of life. Treatment may control the disease, but seldom brings about remission.

Because both of these diseases are rare, there is a general feeling among patients that they are not getting the information they need from the physicians attending their case. This leads to a concern that they may not be receiving the treatment that is most appropriate. This book strives to inform patients and their families of both the usual and the unusual manifestations of GBS and CIDP and some related neuropathies, thereby empowering the patient to ask intelligent and informed questions of their attending physicians. We believe this book contains a unique perspective on Guillain-Barré syndrome since it is written by a physician who was diagnosed with GBS and a neurologist who has spent more than 30 years trying to better understand the disease, teaching patients and physicians about it. We hope that this book is a practical and useful source of information.

Gareth J. Parry, MB, ChB, FRACP
Joel S. Steinberg, MD, PhD

Acknowledgments

We are indebted to Diana Schneider, Edith Barry, and Joseph Hanson of Demos Medical Publishing for their constant encouragement and their seemingly limitless patience when the project lagged behind deadlines. We appreciate the help and advice of our long-time friend and colleague, Dr. David Cornblath, at Johns Hopkins University, who read through the entire manuscript not just once, but twice, and provided invaluable advice regarding content and organization. We also wish to thank the American Academy of Neurology and Dr. Austin Sumner for their recognition of the importance of this topic and for asking us to produce this book.

Most importantly, we would like to express our gratitude to Estelle Benson for her tireless work on behalf of GBS and CIDP patients worldwide through the establishment of the GBS/CIDP Foundation International. We hope that this book will help to further the work of this organization in informing and educating patients and families about these disorders.

GJP
JSS

CHAPTER 1

What Is Guillain-Barré Syndrome?

Gullain-Barre syndrome (GBS) is a type of peripheral neuropathy—Ga condition involving nerves extending into the head, trunk, and limbs. In order to understand GBS, it is first necessary to understand how the nervous system functions.

ORGANIZATION OF THE NERVOUS SYSTEM

The human nervous system consists of the brain and spinal cord, referred to collectively as the *central nervous system* (CNS), and the nerves that extend into the head, trunk, and limbs, known as the *peripheral nervous system.* At the point where the peripheral nerves first emerge from the spinal cord, they are known as *nerve roots* or *radicles.* Damage to a nerve root is called *radiculopathy.* Peripheral nerves consist of bundles of hundreds of individual nerve fibers, each smaller than a human hair. They transmit electrical impulses, allowing the brain to keep in touch with all aspects of bodily function. Sensory nerve fibers send messages from peripheral structures, such as the skin, joints, and bones, to the brain. Motor fibers send

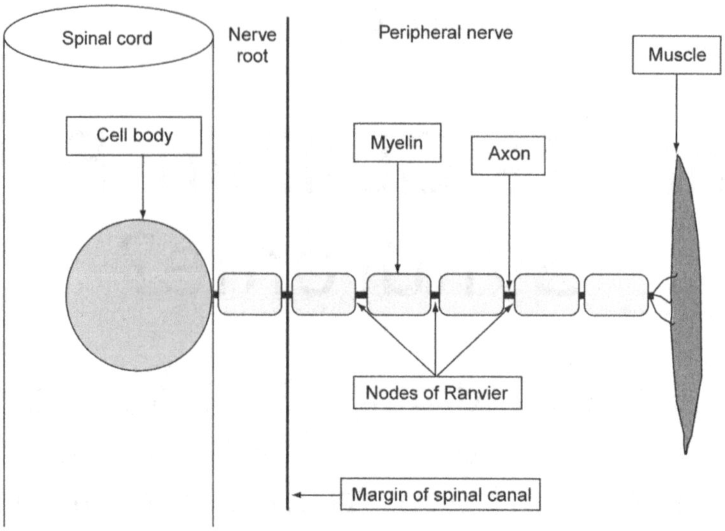

FIGURE 1-1: Schematic representation of the organization of a peripheral motor nerve. The cell body, or motor neuron, lies in the spinal cord. The axon is the nerve cable that connects the spinal cord with the muscle, along which the electrical impulses travel to make the muscle contract. The peripheral nerve where it first emerges from the spinal cord which lies within the spinal canal and is known as the nerve root. When the peripheral nerve emerges from the spinal canal it is known as a spinal nerve. Each spinal nerve merges with many others to form the peripheral nerve. Each motor axon divides into multiple small branches after it enters the muscle, and each branch provides the nerve supply to multiple muscle fibers so that a single motor neuron controls the function of many muscle fibers.

messages from the brain to the muscles. These messages are sent in the form of electrical impulses. Each nerve fiber consists of an electrical cable known as an *axon,* and an insulating sheath known as the *myelin* (Figure 1-1). The myelin sheath is not a continuous structure, but consists of multiple segments of myelin, each separated by a short gap known as the *node of Ranvier.* The node of Ranvier is where the electrical current is generated and renewed.

Peripheral neuropathy—also known as *polyneuropathy* or simply *neuropathy*—is the term used to describe any disorder of peripheral nerves. Peripheral neuropathy that results primarily from the degeneration of axons is known as an *axonal neuropathy. Demyelinating neuropathy* results from degeneration of the myelin. In almost all neuropathies there is a combination of axonal degeneration and demyelination. Peripheral neuropathy that evolves over days to weeks is an *acute* disorder, whereas neuropathy that evolves over months or years is considered *chronic.* Most peripheral neuropathies are chronic disorders.

GUILLAIN-BARRÉ SYNDROME AS A NEUROPATHY

GBS is an *acute* peripheral neuropathy because it evolves over days to weeks. As with other neuropathies, GBS may be axonal, demyelinating, or mixed.

Guillain-Barré syndrome is a type of peripheral neuropathy—a condition involving degeneration of the nerves extending into the head, body, and limbs.

In Europe, North America, and other developed countries, GBS is most commonly a demyelinating neuropathy, and is known as a *cute inflammatory demyelinating polyneuropathy* (AIDP). In this form of GBS, the immune attack is directed against the myelin, causing loss of the myelin sheath and leading to a "short circuit" so that electrical messages cannot travel between the brain and the periphery of the body. There can be secondary damage to the axons in AIDP, but sometimes the primary immune-mediated attack is against the axon itself, causing the electrical cable to degenerate. This is called *axonal GBS,* and it does occur in developed countries, but is uncommon. AIDP is still the most common form of GBS in developing countries, but the axonal form is relatively more common than it is in developed countries. GBS is sometimes called a *polyradiculoneuropathy* because there is a predilection for the demyelination to affect the nerve roots where they first emerge from the spinal cord.

In some cases of axonal GBS, the attack is limited to the motor axons that control muscle activity. This is called *acute motor axonal neuropathy* (AMAN). This form of GBS causes only weakness, with no involvement of sensation. When axonal GBS affects both sensory and motor functions, it is known as *acute motor and sensory axonal neuropathy* (AMSAN). AMSAN is probably a more severe form of AMAN. It is commonly seen as summer outbreaks in children in northern rural China. When there is extensive axonal degeneration, whether the secondary axonal degeneration of AIDP or the primary axonal degeneration of AMAN or AMSAN, recovery is slower and there is a greater likelihood of some residual weakness.

Occasionally, GBS causes paralysis of the eye muscles and loss of balance and coordination. This condition is known as *Miller Fisher syndrome* (MFS), also known as the Fisher syndrome. Thus, GBS is not a single disease, but a group of disorders consisting of AIDP, AMAN, AMSAN, MFS, and other rare variants. Table 1-1 lists the various forms of GBS and their manifestations.

GUILLAIN-BARRÉ SYNDROME AS A DISEASE OF THE IMMUNE SYSTEM

GBS is also an *autoimmune disease.* The immune system is designed to fight invaders from outside the body, mainly viruses and bacteria. It also performs important surveillance for damaged host cells, such as cancer cells. However, for reasons that are only partly understood, the immune system may turn around and attack the body, resulting in autoimmune disease. The immune cells responsible for such an attack are white blood cells known as *lymphocytes.* These cells are involved in inflammation, and they are also known generically as *inflammatory* cells. Thus, one characteristic pathologic hallmark of autoimmune disease is inflammation with lymphocytes. In the more frequent demyelinating form of GBS, the immune system attacks the myelin, resulting in demyelination and inflammation, which can be seen with a microscope. GBS is also unusual in that it evolves acutely, over a period of up to 4 weeks, which is why it is referred to as an acute condition. A similar disorder, which will be discussed separately, differs mainly by virtue of the chronic pace of progression. This type of disorder is referred to as *chronic inflammatory demyelinating polyneuropathy* (CIDP). Both GBS and CIDP have a particular predilection for involvement of the nerve roots, and they are often known as *radiculoneuropathies* rather than simply *neuropathies.* The immune attack is directed against the axon in AMAN and AMSAN.

Table 1-1 Classification of GBS

1. Acute inflammatory demyelinating polyneuropathy (AIDP)

a. Primary damage affects the myelin sheath.

b. Causes acute weakness of limb and breathing muscles.

c. Causes sensory symptoms and signs (numbness, tingling).

2. Acute motor axonal neuropathy (AMAN)

a. Primary damage affects motor axons.

b. Causes acute weakness of limb and breathing muscles.

c. Sensation is normal.

3. Acute motor and sensory axonal neuropathy (AMSAN)

a. Damage affects both motor and sensory axons.

b. Causes acute weakness of limb and breathing muscles.

c. Causes sensory symptoms and signs (numbness, tingling).

4. Miller Fisher syndrome (MFS)

a. Primary site of damage uncertain.

b. Causes acute weakness of eye muscles (ophthalmoplegia)

c. Causes loss of balance and incoordination (ataxia)

d. Causes loss of reflexes (areflexia).

A BRIEF HISTORY OF GUILLAIN-BARRÉ SYNDROME

In 1916, three French neurologists, Guillain, Barré, and Strohl, published their famous account of the condition that now bears the names of the first two physicians. However, recognition of this disorder preceded them by about 80 years, and, in retrospect, several hundred cases of an identical disorder had been described in the intervening period. The earliest known descriptions appeared in the 1830s. In 1834, an English physician, James Wardrop, reported a 35-year-old man who developed numbness that briefly preceded loss of strength. Over 10 days, he lost all of his physical strength except for the ability to turn his head and move his toes. Although there was no comment regarding the man's respiration, it was presumably normal since he survived. Despite sensory symptoms, the sensory examination was normal, as were bowel, bladder, and vital functions. This acute paralytic illness was preceded by diarrhea. Upon treatment by purging, the patient began to recover, and "several years afterward [he was] in the enjoyment of good health, having never had any return of the symptoms." In 1837, a French neurologist from Bordeaux named Ollivier described two people with acutely evolving paralysis. One person developed symptoms after giving birth and died 2 days later. Autopsy failed to reveal any pathologic abnormality of the brain or spinal cord, but the peripheral nerves were not examined. The second person developed severe weakness of all limbs, muscles of the torso, and the respiratory and cranial muscles, and yet made a spontaneous recovery. The recovery of strength in Wardrop's case and in one of Ollivier's was an extraordinary occurrence given the grim prognosis for severe *poliomyelitis* (polio), the usual acute paralytic illness of that era.

General Richard Taylor, the son of the twelfth president of the United States, may have had GBS. In the early 1860s, he developed a fever followed by weakness, but made a complete recovery and resumed his duties for the Confederate cause in the Civil War.

It has been suggested that the well-known illness of President Franklin Delano Roosevelt may have been GBS, not polio, as has been long assumed.

In a paper published in the *Journal of Medical Biography* in 2003, Goldman and associates suggested that the nature of Roosevelt's illness was more consistent with GBS than with poliomyelitis. They evaluated the various features of his illness as recorded in the public record, and concluded that there were more features in common with GBS than with polio. However, this is not a consensus position; most people familiar with GBS feel that his illness was much more typical of polio than GBS. As with all revisions of history, the truth will probably never be known.

In 1859, Jean-Baptiste Octave Landry described a man with weakness that evolved over 8 days from onset to death. He experienced an ill-defined period of muscle cramps and tingling in the limbs preceding paralysis. The muscles of his chest and abdomen were involved, including his diaphragm, resulting in mild respiratory difficulty. There was weakness of the tongue and jaw, and his swallowing was impaired. He experienced mild loss of sensation, and his reflexes were absent. He had rapid heartbeat at rest, his hands and feet were cold despite high seasonal temperature, and he had sphincter weakness. His death was sudden, and may have been due to an irregular heartbeat because there did not appear to have been significant respiratory compromise at the time of death. Thus, all of the classic clinical features of Guillain-Barré syndrome were carefully documented by Landry, who noted that he had seen four other cases and had identified five more from the literature, including the two previously described by Ollivier. Of these 10 cases, only two were fatal. No significant new clinical features were added to this account by Landry until C. Miller Fisher concluded that the syndrome of *ophthalmoplegia, ataxia,* and *areflexia* was a form of Guillain-Barré syndrome.

The 1916 observation and description by Guillain, Barré, and Strohl of "radiculoneuritis with hyperalbuminosis of the cerebrospinal fluid without cellular reaction" were truly original. That is, they noted that the protein in the *cerebrospinal fluid* (CSF) was increased *(hyperalbuminosis)* without an increase in the number of white blood cells. The most common cause of acute weakness at that time was polio, which led to increased numbers of white blood cells in the CSF. It was primarily the CSF findings that led two influential French neurologists, Draganescu and Claudian, to designate the disorder *Guillain-Barré syndrome* in 1927. Andre Strohl was an electrophysiologist who probably contributed the observation that the response of nerves and muscles to electrical stimulation was preserved. It is not entirely clear why Strohl's contribution to the original description was later ignored. It may have been his lack of seniority (he was only 29 years old at the time) or his closer association with physical medicine than with neurology.

Degeneration of peripheral nerves in patients with "Landry's paralysis" was first reported in the late nineteenth century. It was not until then that the concept of peripheral neuropathy as an entity was widely accepted. Early reports did not distinguish between primary and secondary myelin degeneration. The primary demyelinating nature of the common form of the disorder was recognized during the 1950s. In the 1980s, it was confirmed that, in some cases, the primary attack was directed at the axons rather than the myelin. Thus, the term *acute motor axonal neuropathy* was coined. The term *Guillain-Barré syndrome* is now used to designate people who meet the clinical criteria for diagnosis, and they are further defined as having demyelinating or axonal GBS, based on electrophysiologic criteria.

From the earliest reports, it was recognized that the nerves and muscles of people with GBS retain their responses to electrical stimuli. Techniques to study changes in nerve conduction in human neuropathies began to be used regularly in the 1950s. The finding of severe slowing of conduction velocity in GBS was first reported in 1956. The entire spectrum of electrophysiologic changes was reported in detail a few years later. These studies have played a critical role in the diagnosis of GBS ever since.

The greatest single advancement in the treatment of GBS came shortly after the Second World War with the development of artificial ventilation. The subsequent refinement of positive-pressure ventilation and the introduction of intensive care units were responsible for the dramatic fall in mortality during the 1950s. The increased understanding of GBS as an autoimmune process spurred further study of immune therapies in the late 1970s, leading to the widespread use of *plasmapheresis* and, more recently, high-dose intravenous *immunoglobulin.* These are the first treatments available to reliably influence the course of the disease.

The evolution of our appreciation of neuropathy in general, and Guillain-Barré syndrome in particular, has involved some of the most influential neurologists and other physicians of the nineteenth and twentieth centuries, as well as a number of obscure contributors. The dramatic nature of the disease has stimulated interest that is out of proportion to its prevalence. Reasonable expectations for the future include a better understanding of how the disease occurs and the development of more effective and safer treatments.

CHAPTER 2

What Are the Effects of Guillain-Barré Syndrome?

GBS is the common cause of acute paralysis in Western countries because of the virtual elimination of poliomyelitis (polio) with vaccination programs. However, GBS is still a rare disease. Many doctors will never see a case of GBS, which can lead to failure in recognizing it in the early stages. The development of treatments that are the most effective when they are started within two weeks of the onset of symptoms has made it doubly important to recognize the early stages of GBS so appropriate treatment can be started in a timely fashion.

The most common form of GBS in Western countries was described in the early medical literature by Landry, Guillain, and others. This classic form of GBS is characterized primarily by weakness that usually begins in the legs, and then ascends to the upper limbs and cranial area. Weakness often prompts a person with developing GBS to seek medical attention. However, the first symptoms of GBS are often abnormal sensations, usually pins and needles or tingling in the feet and hands. By the time the average patient goes to the doctor, there will usually be some combination of symmetric weakness, usually in an ascending pattern, and abnormal sensation.

MUSCLE WEAKNESS

Weakness is caused by damage to the motor nerves that go from the brain to the muscles and is usually the outstanding clinical feature of GBS. Weakness usually begins in the legs, and is symmetric—meaning it affects both sides of the body equally—although some difference from side to side may be seen. This contrasts with weakness caused by a stroke, which usually affects only one side of the body. In some people, the parts of the limbs farthest from the spinal cord (the *distal* muscles) are the most affected. In others, the muscles located close to the spinal cord (the *proximal* muscles) are weaker. Approximately half of the people affected by GBS have weakness equally in both the proximal and distal muscles. Their thighs, legs, ankles, and feet become uniformly weak, causing the legs to become limp, or flaccid. This is often described as a "rubbery" feeling. Children may say that their legs feel like Jello. Weakness of the legs causes tripping, and difficulty walking, going up and down stairs, or arising from low chairs. As GBS progresses, over days to at most 4 weeks, the weakness typically ascends up the body, involving the hands and arms. This can make it difficult to hold up the arms while shaving, cleaning the teeth, or brushing the hair. Weakness of the hands may cause difficulty holding a comb or toothbrush, or difficulty with fine motor tasks, such as buttoning clothes, writing, or typing.

Muscle weakness is the primary symptom in GBS. It develops rapidly, over days to weeks, and generally affects the legs first. Eventually it may affect all of the muscles, including those that control breathing, speech, and swallowing. Complete paralysis may occasionally occur.

If weakness continues to progress, the breathing, or respiratory, muscles may become involved. About one-fourth of the people afflicted with GBS develop some problems with breathing. The principal muscles of respiration are the *intercostal* muscles, located between the ribs, and the diaphragm, just under the lungs. As the breathing muscles weaken, the person with GBS may be unable to take a normal or deep breath. Coughing may be compromised, and they may pant or take more frequent shallow breaths to compensate for weak muscles. They may complain of a sense of suffocating. People at this stage of GBS may be considered to be simply anxious because many of the symptoms of weak respiratory muscles are similar to those associated with anxiety.

Head and neck muscles can also become weak. These muscles are controlled by a set of nerves called the *cranial* nerves, which come directly off the brain and supply various parts of the head and neck with sensation and strength. Facial weakness is the most common cranial symptom, affecting about one-half of people with GBS, resulting in an inability to smile or fully close the eyes. These symptoms are due to involvement of the seventh cranial nerve. Facial weakness may develop shortly after limb weakness, or it may be the first symptom. It is usually symmetric, but occasionally it may be so asymmetric, with one side of the face drooping more than the other, that the affected person may be thought to have *Bell's palsy.* Weakness of the eye muscles can cause double vision. Difficulty swallowing and handling saliva develops about 15 percent of the time because of involvement of the ninth and tenth cranial nerves. The throat musculature can become weak, compromising integrity of the airway. People so affected may choke on their own secretions and have trouble maintaining an intact airway. These potential complications typically warrant immediate medical attention with an airway tube in order to prevent aspiration of saliva or stomach contents into the lungs. Rarely, tongue weakness may result from damage to the twelfth cranial nerve and affect speech. In extremely severe cases, there may be loss of all voluntary muscle movement and the person will not be able to communicate. This is sometimes called the *locked-in syndrome.* People with this condition may appear to be comatose, yet maintain full awareness of their surroundings.

ABNORMAL SENSATIONS

Although weakness is usually the most prominent feature of GBS, abnormal sensation is often the initial event, occurring hours to days before weakness becomes evident. Sensory symptoms occur in 50 to 70 percent of GBS patients, and can take many forms. Abnormal sensations are called *paresthesias.* If they are particularly unpleasant, they are called *dysesthesias.* Pins and needles or tingling are common examples of paresthesias. People may also complain of numbness or loss of sensation, but this is less common. Typically, these sensations are felt in the parts of the limbs farthest from the spinal cord: the toes, feet, or fingers.

In about 30 percent of GBS patients, there is painful muscle cramping between the shoulder blades or in the lower back or thighs, and the muscles may be tender. Some people experience a sensation of tiny insects crawling over their skin, a condition called *formications.* Some people find this so peculiar that they may be embarrassed to tell their doctor, yet formications are very real. Other sensory illusions may also occur; for example, a sense of vibration, which is probably a variation of paresthesias. There may be a sense of pressure, as if something was forcing them down onto the bed. This may be related to difficulty breathing. Pain is also common in GBS.

Although muscle weakness is the most prominent feature of GBS, abnormal sensations are common. They are often the *first* symptoms experienced by a person who is developing GBS.

Loss of sensation may also occur, but this is usually minor. Some people with GBS may be aware that they cannot feel the sheets normally when they are in bed, or that the temperature of the floor is reduced when they walk with bare feet. Perhaps a more common manifestation of the loss of sensation is ataxia, an imbalance that can occur in any case of GBS. This is particularly prominent in Miller Fisher syndrome. For example, the person may develop a waddling or unsteady, duck-like gait. The unusual gait may reflect weakness of the hip muscles, but also a loss of the ability to sense the position of the limbs without looking at them. The ability to sense limb position is called *proprioception.* Loss of proprioception accounts for the ataxia of Miller Fisher syndrome. Most often, the loss of sensation occurs without the person's awareness but can be detected by neurologic examination. Rarely, there may be a loss of sensation or abnormal sensation with minimal or no weakness.

The loss of reflexes is integral to GBS and is an important manifestation of the involvement of the sensory nerve fibers. A reflex is not really a symptom, and a person with GBS cannot feel reflexes or their loss. However, the loss of reflexes is an important finding that can help make a diagnosis. The reflexes of interest in GBS are the muscle stretch reflexes, which are also called *deep tendon reflexes.* To elicit these reflexes, the tendon of a muscle is tapped with a rubber hammer, which will cause it to suddenly stretch the attached muscle. The stretched muscle briefly and briskly contracts, and then relaxes in an automatic reaction. The knee reflex is perhaps the most well-known *muscle stretch reflex.* When the doctor taps the tendon just below the knee, the attached *quadriceps* muscle in the front of the thigh will suddenly contract, causing the leg to jerk forward.

Absent or diminished muscle stretch reflexes are a major finding in GBS. Indeed, the finding of normal reflexes will typically lead a doctor to strongly doubt GBS and look for another explanation for symptoms. Common sites of testing for muscle stretch reflexes include the knee, the ankle (by tapping the *Achilles tendon* at the back of the ankle), and the arms. Although loss of reflexes is a hallmark of the disease, it may not actually be present at the time of the initial medical assessment. In such a situation, a diagnosis of GBS will likely not be made until weakness is more prominent and the accompanying reflexes are diminished or absent. Repeated examinations may be necessary to help direct the doctor toward a diagnosis of GBS.

PAIN IN GUILLAIN-BARRÉ SYNDROME

GBS is a disorder in which the dramatic nature of the paralysis overshadows all other features. Pain is an integral part of the disease, but sometimes it is not given sufficient attention. In some studies, pain has been reported in more than 80 percent of people with GBS. It is frequently underappreciated and undertreated by doctors, especially in the intensive care unit (ICU), where people with GBS may not be able to communicate about their pain. They may have been incorrectly told that they do *not* have pain because pain does not occur in GBS. The pain of GBS can occur during the acute phase of the illness, and may even predate the onset of weakness. Pain can also occur during recovery and rehabilitation. This section covers only the pain that occurs during the acute illness. Pain occurring during rehabilitation will be discussed in a later section.

Pain may be the first symptom of GBS, or it may develop together with weakness. It is generally proportional to the severity of the weakness; that is, severe pain is seen mainly in people with severe weakness. Typically, the pain of GBS is located in the region of the spine and the upper parts of the limbs, including pain between the shoulder blades, in the lower back and buttocks, or around the hips and shoulders. This early pain is often difficult to describe, but it tends to have an aching or cramping quality. There may be stabs of pain with movement that may not be at one clearly localized point, but rather somewhat diffuse. It may seem to be deep in the body rather than on the surface. Fortunately, this type of pain is usually no more than a nuisance. Occasionally, it may be severe, particularly in people on ventilators who have rapidly progressive and severe paralysis, and they should be asked specifically if they are experiencing pain. This is the most neglected type of pain seen in GBS because the doctor is concentrating on the life-threatening aspects of the disease. Severe pain may cause dangerous heart irregularities and changes in blood pressure.

Pain is a common early feature of GBS, but it is frequently overlooked. It is important to ask people with GBS whether they are experiencing pain because they may have difficulty communicating.

Pain in the acute phase of GBS is called *nociceptive* pain, not *neuropathic* pain. Nociceptive pain is the type of pain that warns us of tissue damage; irreparable damage might occur if it did not hurt to walk on a broken leg. The perception of pain offers important protection against injury. By contrast, neuropathic pain is pain that arises from damaged nerve fibers. It serves no useful protective function. Neuropathic pain occurs during recovery from the acute phase of GBS.

It is important to distinguish between nociceptive and neuropathic pain because they require different treatments. Nociceptive pain is best treated with simple painkillers *(analgesics).* If the pain is mild, nonsteroidal, anti-inflammatory drugs (NSAIDs), such as aspirin, acetaminophen (Tylenol®), ibuprofen (Advil® or Motrin®), and naproxen (Naprosyn® or Aleve®, may be all that is needed. More severe pain can be treated with oral narcotics, such as codeine, meperidine (Demerol®, oxycodone (Oxycontin®, or hydrocodone (Vicodin®. Often, narcotics are used in combination with NSAIDs, most commonly acetaminophen with codeine. If medication cannot be swallowed safely, analgesics can be given by injection, usually intravenously. There is no need for people with GBS to suffer pain, and doctors should not hesitate to use powerful narcotic analgesics if necessary. However, care must be taken when prescribing narcotics for people with GBS, who may have reduced respiratory function, because narcotics can cause respiratory failure. There is little cause for concern if the person is already on a ventilator. Respiratory function needs to be very closely monitored so that mechanical ventilation can be used if necessary. Some people prefer to tolerate pain rather than risk going on a ventilator, but they need to be counseled regarding the risks and benefits. Pain during the acute phase of GBS may resolve rapidly during treatment.

It is also important to realize that immobility causes pain, or at least discomfort. Lying in one position can become very uncomfortable. This can be alleviated by frequent turning and passive movement of paralyzed limbs, which makes experienced, high-quality nursing care important.

THE EFFECTS OF AUTONOMIC NERVE INVOLVEMENT

The *autonomic nerves* are a group of peripheral nerves, located throughout the body, that automatically regulate the internal organs of the body. The effects of damage to these nerves are more readily recognized by the doctor than by the person with GBS. Autonomic symptoms are shown in Table 2-1.

Table 2-1 Autonomic Symptoms Occurring During the Course of GBS

- Difficulty urinating or inability to void (urinary retention)
- Constipation or paralyzed bowel (paralytic ileus)
- Lightheadedness or fainting (syncope) upon arising caused by low blood pressure
- Pounding headache from elevated blood pressure
- Palpitations of the heart from a rapid or irregular heart beat
- Confusion or seizures caused by low blood salt (sodium) level

- Increased sweating
- Bluish discoloration and cold temperature of the hands and feet resulting from abnormal nervous system control of blood flow to the limbs (vasomotor instability)

Abnormalities of autonomic function tend to be worse in people with severe weakness, including those who require breathing support. Most people with GBS experience some autonomic nerve damage, which is usually only apparent to the examining doctor. The most common effect is an increased heart rate at rest. On rare occasions, there may be serious irregularities of the heart rhythm, requiring medical treatment or even a temporary pacemaker. Wide fluctuations of blood pressure from very high to very low can also occur, but care must be exercised in treating elevated blood pressure because people with GBS are very sensitive to the drugs administered in the ICU for high blood pressure. These autonomic cardiac abnormalities can be exacerbated by pain, so aggressive pain management is essential. Low blood pressure may not be noticed until the person is able to get out of bed. The upright position results in a sometimes dramatic fall in blood pressure, a condition known as *orthostatic hypotension.* People in whom the disease is severe enough to necessitate care in the ICU will often have a bladder catheter, and will not be aware of difficulty with urination. Similarly, lack of bowel movements may simply be attributed to reduced food intake and immobility.

GBS may affect the autonomic nerves that control internal organs, as well as those that control motor and sensory functions. Minor disturbances of heart rhythm are common and occasionally severe. There may also be changes in blood pressure, abnormal sweating, constipation, and urine retention.

CHILDREN WITH GUILLAIN-BARRÉ SYNDROME

There are no substantive differences in the way that GBS affects children compared with adults. The initial symptoms are pain and tingling, but these are often unrecognized. Their significance may be unappreciated because the child may not articulate accurately their symptoms. Pain may cause irritability that is thought to be the result of a nonspecific illness, particularly if the child has had a virus recently. This can lead to a slight delay in diagnosis, but usually not more than 24 hours, as it will quickly become clear that something is seriously wrong once weakness develops. The weakness may manifest primarily as a problem with running or a tendency to fall or drop things. The distribution of weakness and its severity is the same for children and adults. Children are no more or less likely to develop cranial nerve involvement or respiratory failure. Children and young adults recover from GBS better than older adults. Useful information about the nuances of dealing with childhood GBS can be obtained from Patricia Schardt's writings[1] about dealing with her daughter Melissa's 5-year experience with CIDP, a chronic variant of GBS.

One of the major issues facing the family of a child with GBS is the fear of a poor recovery. A cautiously optimistic approach is important for both adults and children. Personal attention in the hospital and frequent visits from family members and friends will be necessary. They should bring mementos from home, such as a favorite toy or piece of clothing. A child with a serious illness inevitably puts tremendous strain on the family, including the fear of death, disability, and the unknown. The efforts of a caring parent to provide love and support to a child who has GBS—while simultaneously trying to give equal attention to other members of the family and retain a semblance of normality at home and work—inevitably generates anxiety, frustration, anger, fatigue, and fear. The following guidelines may help families deal with a child's illness:

---

1 A publication of the GBS/CIDP Foundation International, Caring For a Child with GBS.

Guidelines for the Family of a Child with GBS

- Accept assistance from friends and extended family when offered, and do not hesitate to ask for support. Even if help is needed only with small chores, such as picking up the other children from school, it will help ease the burden.
- Healthy siblings of children with GBS usually have conflicting emotions. They are concerned and want to help, but they may feel guilty that they are healthy while their sibling is not. They may also resent the attention that the child with GBS receives. It is important to educate the other family members about GBS—it is no one's fault; bad things happen to good people; and most people recover, but it may take some time.
- Explain that every attempt will be made to keep family life as normal as possible, but that the family member with GBS will need extra attention.
- Let the healthy siblings participate in care of the sibling with GBS as much as they can, including frequent visits to the hospital and assisting with therapy or homework.
- Teenagers may resent the intrusion on their social life. They may be embarrassed to talk about the family member with GBS or push a wheelchair. This is the time to be empathetic to their needs, but also to educate them about the responsibility and the sense of accomplishment that can be

gained from helping another person in need—as that person would likely do for them if the situation were reversed.

- Parents should spend some one-on-one quality time with each healthy sibling in order to assure them that the world does not exclusively revolve around the child who has GBS. The doctors, nurses, and therapists will do the best they can to provide medical care. The role of the family is to support the child with GBS and each other.
- When the child comes home from the hospital, but is still in outpatient rehabilitation and has not yet gone back to school, do not let illness be an excuse for them to be resentful or overly demanding. Fatigue is to be expected, and the child's household responsibilities should be adjusted accordingly. Fatigue in GBS is very real, and the recovering child may have to take naps or rest during the day. Making judgments about whether the child is legitimately exhausted or merely being manipulative can be challenging. This can test parenting skills.

EMOTIONAL ISSUES

Although the emotional impact of GBS usually begins with the initial onset of the disease, emotional issues are not addressed in most neurology and other medical books. The importance of emotional issues cannot be overstated, as they play a central role in the ability of the family to deal with the illness.

The importance of emotional issues cannot be overstated, as they play a central role in the ability of the family to deal with the illness.

This illness takes a toll from the beginning—not just on the person with GBS, but the rest of the family as well. The initial symptoms of tingling or pain, even before weakness develops, often leave the person with GBS and family puzzled and concerned. This illness usually affects previously healthy individuals, who have probably never experienced symptoms of this type before. If medical attention is sought at this early stage, it is not uncommon for the examining doctor to suspect anxiety or stress as the cause of symptoms rather than a physical disorder. This adds to the confusion, frustration, and worry. Most people have never even heard of GBS, so when the diagnosis is finally made they become even more confused. They may wonder how the disorder happened, what they did to deserve it, and what the future has in store. The situation can be frightening, and given the fact that progressive weakness is likely, respiratory failure is possible, and the final outcome is unpredictable, their fears are grounded in reality. Caregivers and the person with GBS should keep in mind that the outcome is usually good. Yes, there will be loss of muscle control, and maybe even an inability to breathe without support, but it helps if everyone involved can see past the current difficulties and remember there is the likelihood of eventual recovery. Caregivers will need to reassess their priorities after the diagnosis of GBS in a family member, perhaps putting some activities on hold so they can be supportive.

Emotional support should not be the responsibility of only one person, although the closest relative usually bears the brunt of the supporting role. Hopefully, emotional support efforts will involve the participation of a team that includes a receptive patient, supportive family and friends, and caring medical professionals. Most newly-diagnosed people are placed in an ICU or comparable part of the hospital in order to monitor their vital signs closely, including breathing, heart rate, and blood pressure. This situation opens up a whole set of emotional issues that add to the aggravation of the diagnosis of a rare, paralyzing disorder. Visiting hours in the ICU are limited, and medical personnel may or may not be friendly or informative. Fear can set in, perhaps magnified by explanations being given in confusing medical jargon. The early stages of GBS can be frightening, and emotional support is especially important at this time.

Many people with GBS have been previously healthy. They are seldom emotionally prepared for illness, especially one that appears to be catastrophic. Realizing they are paralyzed and that they are attached to intravenous lines, a bladder catheter, and a heart monitor can be extremely upsetting. Brushing their teeth, feeding themselves, or scratching an itch can become impossible. If a breathing machine is required, the inability to communicate and the resulting sense of isolation can become frustrating. Feelings of helplessness and hopelessness, fear of death, the possibility of permanent disability, and the loss of independence and income can be overwhelming. It is helpful for both the person with GBS and their family to keep in mind that most people recover and ultimately resume a normal life.

It is helpful for both the person with GBS and the family to keep in mind that most people recover and ultimately resume a normal life.

One valuable strategy for helping to alleviate the fear of permanent disability is to arrange for visits from people who have had GBS and recovered. The GBS/CIDP Foundation International has local chapters in many cities, and many recovered people are only too happy to help an affected individual through this difficult illness.

People with a serious illness typically go through a series of emotional reactions before finally accepting their situation:

- *Disbelief and denial:* "This can't be happening to me. I must have a more common, treatable disease. Maybe the doctor made the wrong diagnosis."
- *Fear:* "What will happen to me and my family? How long will I be sick? Can I handle this?"

- *Anger:* "Why did this happen to me? What did I do to deserve GBS?"
- *Bargaining:* "If I get better quickly, get off the respirator, or really have a more benign disease, in return I will...."
- *Frustration:* "I'm fed-up with being in the hospital and want to go home. I'm tired of needing to wait for others to help me. I don't want to be dependent on others."
- *Depression:* "I feel terrible. I'll never get better. I must deserve to be punished. I'm worn out. I can't put up with this any longer."
- *Acceptance:* "I'll do the best I can. Things could be worse. Thank goodness I'm still alive."

How to Reduce Emotional Stress in the ICU

People with GBS, especially those in an ICU or on a ventilator, may benefit from the following suggestions:

Explain the disorder. Early in the hospital stay, GBS should be explained clearly to everyone involved, including the relatively good chance for recovery. If family, friends, and medical personnel understand the disease, they can present a more optimistic outlook to the person with GBS.

Communication cards. The person on a respirator may feel less frustrated if a method for communicating with others is provided. The GBS/CIDP Foundation can provide a bound set of "Communication Cards." (see Resources). These cards state in large print the common problems and questions that may arise. A nurse or family member can use the cards to communicate with the patient by pointing to various items and getting a "yes" or "no" head nod or eye movement response. Remember, people on respirators can still hear, feel, and think.

Explain activities. Explanations by nurses, respiratory therapists, physical therapists, and other medical attendants regarding procedures and other standard hospital activities will help alleviate anxiety when unfamiliar procedures are performed, especially painful ones.

Frequent visits. The presence of family and friends shows caring and provides moral support. Develop a rotation among visitors, perhaps assigning several people a particular day of the week to visit, so the person with GBS can always depend on having a loved nearby.

Keep track of time. A clock, electric calendar, radio, and night light can help keep track of day and night, maintain awareness of the outside world, improve orientation, and minimize confusion. This is especially important in windowless ICUs.

Pain. Explain to the person with GBS that pain and abnormal sensations are common and can be controlled.

Emotional expression. Allowing the person with GBS to express their emotions, including anger, frustration, and fear, will help them deal with their feelings.

Get involved. Reading get well cards and discussing family events can the reduce sense of isolation, which is common during a prolonged hospital stay.

Assist the nurses. Close family members can offer to help with grooming. Busy nurses and aides usually welcome this type of assistance.

Contact doctor. Designate a central figure to call for explanations regarding status and care plans. This should be an accessible person with good bedside rapport, ideally a neurologist with a good understanding of the disease and its management. In some hospitals, this may be the internist. Once the person with GBS has been transferred to a rehabilitation center, a physiatrist will usually take the lead in providing care.

Speak to care providers. Learn the names of the care team members and their roles. Remember, it is not just the doctors who are involved in care. The nurses, physical and occupational therapists, and aides are important in caring for the person with GBS. Once you learn who does what, you can start to ask informed questions and get helpful answers. For example, ask the physical therapist or nurse about how the person is being positioned on the bed in order to reduce the risk of bedsores.

Volunteer. Observe the various therapists as they provide range of motion and other exercises. Offer to assist when a therapist is not available, thereby contributing to your loved one's recovery.

Former patient visits. As stated above, a visit from someone who has had GBS and recovered can provide an excellent boost, especially during the acute stage in the ICU.

Diary. Keep a diary highlighting important events on the road to recovery. As your loved one improves, you will have something to reinforce the fact that progress is being made.

Reassurance. Reassure the patient that most people with GBS have a good recovery. Let them know that everyone involved, including doctors, nurses, therapists, family, and friends, will do all they can to help them recover.

This illness can sometimes cause severe emotional reactions. Paying attention to the person with GBS, and not just the disease, is critical in helping to alleviate negative feelings.

Negative reactions. Expect negative reactions. Sometimes people with GBS are angry, depressed, and worried. Guide them in taking an active role in their recovery if possible.

DIFFICULTIES IN MAKING AN EARLY DIAGNOSIS

Weakness is the preeminent feature of GBS, and this should make the diagnosis easy. Indeed, in the majority of new GBS cases, weakness is an obviously new event, causing the person experiencing the weakness to go to the doctor, and asking him or her to look for an explanation. However, individual reports indicate that weakness is not always appreciated as a new event that signals the doctor to look for a new medical problem. This potential dilemma can make the diagnosis of GBS challenging, or even suspect. Weakness may be attributed to the aftereffects of an antecedent event. For example, severe diarrhea or an influenzatype illness can often leave a person with a lack of stamina. Similarly, people undergoing major surgery, and needing artificial ventilation for a period of time afterward, may have difficulty being weaned from the respirator. This may be attributed to the effects of the surgery itself, and new neurologic findings may not be recognized. In such situations, the appearance of new weakness combined with loss of reflexes should lead to a suspicion of GBS. A lumbar puncture and electrodiagnostic studies can then confirm the diagnosis.

Recognizing weakness as a new event, rather than as part of a triggering viral illness, can be particularly challenging in children, who develop infections more frequently than adults and are more often expected to use rest as a treatment. Identifying weakness from GBS as distinct from the weakness and fatigue of an infection may not be easy. The ability of children to verbalize their symptoms may be limited because their vocabulary skills may not be sufficiently developed. Sometimes, an astute parent, rather than the doctor, ultimately recognizes an unusual pattern of weakness and signals concern about a newly evolving neurologic problem.

As many as 70 percent of individuals with possible GBS consult the doctor initially with purely sensory features, such as pain, tingling, or numbness; however, anxiety or even malingering may be suspected. Tingling can reflect disorders other than GBS, including hyperventilation caused by anxiety, pinched median nerve in the wrist from *carpal tunnel syndrome,* foot numbness as a result of pinched nerves in the back, and low back pain from arthritis. The key to arriving at a diagnosis of GBS is reevaluation over a period of several days in order to document the development of weakness and the loss of deep tendon reflexes.

GBS is usually easy to diagnose once weakness develops, although it is best to make the diagnosis *before* there is overt weakness. GBS should be considered in any person who develops new neurologic symptoms following an infection, and strongly suspected if there is the triad of weakness, abnormal sensation, and absent reflexes.

DISEASES THAT RESEMBLE GUILLAIN-BARRÉ SYNDROME

Although many people with GBS complain about the delay in diagnosis, it is probably more likely that other conditions are misdiagnosed as GBS. Some of the disorders that may be mistaken for GBS are listed below.

Poliomyelitis

Poliomyelitis (polio) has been largely eliminated in Western countries, but it remains a scourge in the developing countries. Although occasional cases still occur in North America and other developed countries, most of them are in older, nonvaccinated individuals who have been exposed to recently vaccinated infants.

The polio virus enters the body through the digestive tract. The first sign of infection is usually *gastroenteritis* (food poisoning) with mild fever, but this may be so mild that it is not recognized. After the initial illness, there is usually temporary improvement followed by muscle pain and weakness. Polio differs from GBS in that the weakness of polio is usually asymmetrical, and may even affect only one limb. Sensory symptoms are common, but there are usually no objective sensory abnormalities. Autonomic involvement may also be seen. Cases of polio with sensory and autonomic signs and symptoms are particularly likely to be mistaken for GBS in Western countries. Polio reaches its nadir within 2 to 4 weeks, and complete or partial functional recovery begins slowly thereafter. The degree of recovery is generally proportional to the weakness. For example, people with severe weakness make a poor recovery. Also, the degree of recovery in polio is usually less than in GBS at a similar level of weakness. Vaccine-associated polio tends to be less severe. It may be diagnosed late or missed completely, although severe paralysis has been reported in rare instances.

It is easy to see that the occurrence of an acutely evolving paralysis appearing 10 to 14 days after an episode of gastroenteritis and sometimes associated with back pain and sensory and autonomic symptoms and signs can lead to the mistaken diagnosis of GBS, particularly in Western countries where polio is now rare. Conversely, some cases of GBS are undoubtedly sometimes missed in areas where polio is still common.

West Nile Virus

West Nile virus is a relatively new viral infection that can cause an acutely evolving paralysis. This virus entered the United States through New York and has spread as far as the West Coast. It is transmitted by mosquitoes, so it is exclusively a disease of the warm weather months. Most people who contract West Nile fever experience nothing more than a fever and a general feeling of malaise. It sometimes causes inflammation of the brain *(encephalitis),* leading to headache, mental confusion, and seizures. Even less commonly, it can cause acute paralysis. People with acute paralysis often also have encephalitis, but some cases of paralysis have occurred without encephalitis. The neurologic picture closely resembles polio, and several early reports mistakenly identified West Nile fever as GBS.

An examination of the cerebrospinal fluid (CSF) is critical in distinguishing polio and West Nile viral infections from GBS. The protein concentration is usually normal in viral infections, but there is an increase in the number of inflammatory cells. In contrast, the classic feature of GBS is increased protein concentration with no inflammation. Nerve conduction studies can also help to distinguish between paralysis from viral infections and from GBS. Most cases of GBS are characterized by demyelination, whereas viral infections cause motor nerve cell degeneration (see Chapter 3 for details).

Tick Paralysis

Tick paralysis, as the name indicates, is an acute paralytic illness resulting from a toxin in the saliva of a tick. This toxin is injected into the human body while the tick is feeding. The clinical picture is very similar to GBS, and the correct diagnosis is unlikely to be made unless the tick is found and tested. Ticks are most often found on the scalp in children, more commonly in girls. Ticks are difficult to find without shaving the child's head because they are concealed by hair.

Tick paralysis is seen in many different geographic areas and with several different species of ticks. In North America, tick paralysis is most commonly seen in the northwestern United States and in Canada. However, cases have been reported from eastern and southern states and from the southern Midwest. Tick paralysis is also seen in Australia, Africa, and parts of Asia, but not in Central or South America. The tick that causes tick paralysis is not the same as the one that causes *Lyme disease* nor is it caused by the common wood tick found in many parts of the country.

Neurologic symptoms generally begin 3 to 5 days after the tick becomes attached. The earliest symptoms are fatigue, irritability, tingling sensations, and loss of coordination. These symptoms are followed within a few days by weakness, which develops over a period of hours—much more rapidly than the weakness of GBS. Equally rapid improvement occurs once the tick is *completely* removed. Failure to improve is usually due to incomplete removal of the tick, or to a second, undetected tick. CSF protein is not elevated in tick paralysis, providing an important clue to the correct diagnosis. Nerve conduction studies also are helpful in distinguishing tick paralysis from GBS because there are none of the features that are so characteristic of GBS.

Toxic Neuropathies

Acute poisoning with arsenic or thallium can cause gastrointestinal symptoms, followed by acute weakness and sensory symptoms 2 to 3 weeks later. As in GBS, the CSF protein is often elevated without inflammation. Initially, electrodiagnostic studies results may superficially resemble GBS, but there is usually more axonal degeneration and more sensory involvement in toxic neuropathies. The organophosphate compounds that are commonly used as pesticides can also cause an acute neuropathy resembling GBS. The intoxication is caused by massive accidental exposure in all of these cases. A history is easily obtained; however, concealed poisoning with homicidal or suicidal intent may present diagnostic challenges. People often ask whether GBS can be caused by exposure to toxins in the environment, but there is no evidence of this.

Chronic Inflammatory Demyelinating Polyneuropathy (CIDP)

This chronic disorder, which is described in more detail in Chapter 9, may occasionally have an acute presentation. In this case, there is no reliable way to distinguish between GBS and CIDP, although even in the most acute presentation of CIDP, the evolution is somewhat slower than GBS. The clinical features may be otherwise identical. The CSF protein may be elevated and the electrodiagnostic features may be identical. The person can be treated with the usual measures and may recover, and the correct diagnosis can be reached later when a relapse occurs.

Transverse Myelitis

The authors have met a number of people at support group meetings who almost certainly had inflammation of the spinal cord *(transverse myelitis)* rather than GBS. Weakness is usually confined to the legs in transverse myelitis, and there will be prominent sensory loss and loss of bowel and bladder control. These features may also be seen in GBS but are rare. Loss of sensation in the torso is one important characteristic of transverse myelitis that can help distinguish it from GBS. In addition, reflexes are not usually absent in transverse myelitis. In fact, after 1 to 2 weeks, the reflexes are increased and muscle stiffness *(spasticity)* develops. The correct diagnosis becomes obvious at this point. However, during the first few days it can be difficult to distinguish between these two disorders.

Hysterical Paralysis

Hysterical paralysis is rare, and is seldom confused with GBS. More commonly, GBS is erroneously diagnosed as hysteria early in the evolution of the illness. Paresthesias may be attributed to hyperventilation, and early proximal weakness may result in disturbance of gait before overt weakness can be detected by formal strength testing. The confusion may be compounded by the occasional GBS patient in whom reflexes are preserved early in the course of the disease. Obviously, such confusion could be fatal to someone who develops autonomic or respiratory problems in an inappropriate setting. It is always better to err on the side of safety, and admit people with acute sensory symptoms or weakness into the hospital for monitoring until a definitive diagnosis is established.

GBS is the most common cause of acutely evolving paralysis seen in Western countries. However, there are a number of other disorders that may resemble GBS sufficiently closely that an incorrect diagnosis can be made.

CASE SUMMARIES

The following summaries of actual cases illustrate what can happen to someone who develops GBS, and the varying degrees of recovery.

Case One

On Monday morning, January 5, 1981, Mr. C.S, a 40-year-old industrial materials salesman, had just completed a 10-day stint at work, which included a mixture of office activities and on-the-road selling. At about 8:45A.M., he noticed tingling in his fingertips as he related the highlights of the week to his wife. "That's odd," he thought. "It makes no sense." The tingling lasted a few minutes and then faded away. The next morning, he noticed he needed to hold the handrail in order to pull his body up the stairs. He almost fell over when he arrived at the office, and his business partner thought he probably had the flu and offered to drive him home. On the way, Mr. C.S. started thinking about his unusual situation. Normally, he was a strong person—able to climb ropes in high school with only his bare hands—but now he felt like a whipped pup that was passively letting someone else drive the car. Over the next day and a half, his wife noticed that he walked like a waddling duck and had even more difficulty climbing the stairs. "You're walking strangely," she said, but he ignored her comment.

Then, at 2:00A.M. on Thursday, he became aware that his gums were tingling. "This is really peculiar," he thought. "It's time to see a doctor." He called his regular doctor and a neurologist. He was at the doctor's office sitting on the examination table by 10:00A.M. He had no reflexes; his hip and shoulder muscles were weak; there was a hint of speech changes (his words were not coming out clearly); and abnormalities were found on the nerve conduction study in his muscles when the doctor stimulated the nerve supply in his legs.

The neurologist asked him if he had experienced a recent illness. Mr. C.S. said he had not, but then his wife commented that he had experienced a mild sore throat about a week before. The neurologist said his illness was most likely GBS. A head tomographic (CT) scan was taken, and it was normal. While walking to the car in the doctor's driveway, he slipped on ice and could not get up by himself. His wife and the neurologist helped him, and then she drove him to the hospital where he was admitted into the ICU. (It was not really very bothersome.) His blood was drawn, a chest x-ray was taken, he was hooked up to a heart monitor, and his lungs were checked, and they seemed a bit congested, considering that he did not smoke. An IV line was started, and he was given mini-nebulizer breathing treatments to try to keep his lungs clear.

This series of events had unfolded quickly. Mr. C.S. had no idea what was going to happen next. He and his wife had always been healthy. They had two small children, a new home, and the expectation of a long, healthy life ahead of them, but what did the future hold now? Then they found out that he did *not* need a respirator because his lungs began to clear. He developed more left than right facial drooping, and he had resting blood pressure elevation and rapid heart rate, for which he was given propanolol (Inderal®).

Later, at the rehabilitation hospital, Mr. C.S. learned to walk again—first in the pool, so his weak legs could go through the motions of walking with the support of water, then mat exercises, and eventually he graduated to the parallel bars. He was discharged to a day hospital, but he slept at home and took wheelchair van trips to the hospital for intensive therapy. He returned to work after about 3 months, but only for 1 hour a day, because fatigue would hit. Six months later, he was working full time and could run a bit. He still could not walk more than a block before fatigue would hit and he would have to sit down or collapse. However, his fatigue was gone about 6 to 12 months later. Occasional tingling of his right little finger waned slowly over about 5 years.

Case Two

Mrs. S.B., aged 45 years, had a busy life raising two daughters; one was in high school and one was in college. On the Monday morning after Thanksgiving, December 1, 1980, she noticed her toe was tingling. "That's unusual," she thought. "I wonder what's going on." When she ate breakfast, the orange juice burned her tongue and lips. It was 7:00A.M. After breakfast, while driving, her foot pressed the accelerator and she felt her foot tingle again. Her fingers were tingling too. She drove to her daughter's school, and as usual walked down the corridor to the volunteers' desk. The walk seemed to take longer than usual and was more of an effort. Mrs. S.B. sat down at the desk with a sense of relief, but a telephone call for a teacher forced her to walk down the hall again. This time it was a real effort. She barely made it to the faculty lounge to summon the teacher and then back to the volunteers' desk. "It's time to call the doctor," she thought.

Mrs. S.B.'s husband picked her up and took her to her doctor. The examination showed nothing. Her husband recalled that she had experienced an intestinal virus the week before. She went home, planning to rest and drink lots of liquid, as recommended by her doctor. The evening passed uneventfully; she was able to use the stairs without difficulty. The next morning, she shuffled to the bathroom for a drink of water, but found that she could not swallow. So, it was off to the hospital and through the admission process. There were many forms to sign, and as she sat with her pen poised midair, she found she could not write. She was in a room by 11A.M. Her blood pressure was taken and blood was drawn, but all of the tests said she was okay. A neurologic consultation was planned by the family internist. The neurologist appeared at 7P.M. He discovered that her reflexes were okay. He offered several diagnoses to consider: multiple sclerosis, myasthenia gravis, and Guillain-Barré syndrome. Additional tests were necessary and she was transferred to the intensive care unit (ICU).

Over the next several days her condition worsened and her husband received a call from the internist with the diagnosis of GBS. He had read about it and learned that GBS often follows an infection, causes paralysis, usually starts in the legs, and can move up the body quickly.

Later that day, a breathing tube was placed through Mrs. S.B.'s nose and down her throat and she was connected to the respirator. She awoke hours later with a limp neck. She could still blink or twitch her mouth to communicate. The next day, the twitch was gone. She was now full of tubes and lines: feeding tube, intravenous line, respirator, bladder catheter, sensors for her heart beat, and pulse oximetry to assure that she was getting enough oxygen.

After 4.5 months Mrs. S.B. was removed from the respirator. She was able to stand for the first time a month after that, and she finally went home about a year after she had entered the hospital. Six months later, she was able to handle much of her personal care and dress herself, and she no longer required a home nurse. A gradual recovery continued over many years.

Case Three

K.P., a 24-year-old auto mechanic, was changing a tire when he noticed some low back aches and difficulty in rising. The tire was heavy and he assumed the discomfort was temporary as he continued working. However, the next morning he had trouble getting out of bed and had to hold on to the railing to walk down the stairs. This was so unusual for this robust man that he called his doctor. An examination revealed a waddling gait and no knee or other reflexes. His doctor recalled seeing a case of GBS during training and was concerned because the patient recalled a brief episode of diarrhea during the last week. He was immediately admitted to the hospital and placed in a bed with a heart monitor, and consultation was tendered to the neurologist. Various blood tests and other studies were performed. Most were normal, including a CAT scan of the brain. The neurologist confirmed the primary physician's exam findings and noted leg weakness with a near fall upon attempting to stand. Finger and grip strength were mildly impaired. Spinal fluid was clear, with elevated protein and no cells. Electrical testing of the legs showed nerve conduction slowing supportive of demyelination. A 5-day course of high dose immune globulins was initiated. Physical and occupation therapy and rehabilitation consults were ordered. By day 8 of the patient's stay, he could readily stand, but was shaky upon trying to take a step.

During the next two weeks of therapy in the hospital's acute rehabilitation unit, his gait and walking endurance progressively improved. He maintained good use of his arms and a firm grip, but heavy lifting was still tiring. Plans were made for a home therapy program with a therapist visiting 3 times a week. Within two more weeks he was able to walk around the block and lift a heavy suitcase. He returned to work without problems.

UNUSUAL FORMS OF GUILLAIN-BARRÉ SYNDROME

Although most cases of GBS follow the classic sequence of paralysis ascending from the legs to the upper parts of the body, there are atypical forms that may lead to diagnostic confusion.

Miller Fisher Syndrome (MFS)

In 1956, Dr. C. Miller Fisher described a syndrome that included ataxia, areflexia, and ophthalmoplegia. He suggested that it was a variant of GBS. *Ataxia* is loss of coordination and balance, mainly affecting walking. There may also be clumsiness of the arms. *Ophthalmoplegia* involves weakness of the muscles around the eyes, causing double vision *(diplopia)* and droopy eyelids *(ptosis).* The reaction of the pupil to shining a bright light in the eye may also be affected. The combination of diplopia and ataxia makes walking particularly hazardous, and there is a substantial risk of falls. When a person with MFS is examined, there is loss of the muscle reflexes *(areflexia)* when the tendons in the ankles, knees, and arms are tapped. Other cranial nerves may also be involved, causing facial weakness, difficulty swallowing, and slurred speech. These effects are usually mild. There may also be mild weakness of limb muscles. Some affected people may progress from an initially pure MFS to a more generalized GBS, possibly including respiratory failure, but this is very uncommon. Nonetheless, people with MFS should be admitted to the hospital for observation in order to ensure that the illness remains restricted to the cranial area. Symptoms often come on a week or two after some kind of infectious illness, as in a typical case of GBS. MFS progresses for 1 to 2 weeks, but occasionally for as long as 4 weeks, then stabilizes and steadily improves. Most people fully recover and are back to normal within 2 to 3 months, although some have mild residual ataxia for longer. Diplopia and ptosis almost always completely resolve.

Most cases of GBS result from antibodies attacking the myelin sheath of the peripheral nerves;

occasionally the axon is the primary target. Recent research has shown that MFS is very strongly associated with antibodies to a component of the myelin sheath known as *GQ1b.* Over 90 percent of the people with MFS have these antibodies. MFS makes up about 5 percent of the cases of GBS in most countries, but about 25 percent in Japan. The unusually high incidence of MFS in Japan suggests that some populations are genetically more likely to develop GQ1b antibodies in response to a bacterial or viral infection.

Sensory GBS

The onset of weakness in people with GBS is often preceded by sensory symptoms, such as tingling and a feeling of numbness. When weakness develops, it is so much more dramatic than these minor sensory symptoms that they are often forgotten. Very rarely, weakness does *not* develop, and GBS is purely sensory in its manifestations. In this case, reflexes are always diminished or absent. Some people have problems with balance, which occurs along with the other sensory symptoms despite having normal strength. Unlike weakness, which almost always affects both the proximal and distal muscles, sensory symptoms are usually confined to the hands and feet. Electrodiagnostic studies almost always show abnormal conduction in motor nerves, even when no weakness is found.

Bulbar GBS

Rarely, GBS may begin in the muscles around the face and throat, causing difficulty swallowing and slurred speech. People with bulbar GBS may also have difficulty chewing and weakness of the facial muscles. Occasionally, when facial weakness starts on one side, the affected person may be thought to have Bell's palsy—until the weakness spreads to other muscles. Weakness in this form of GBS usually descends to involve the limbs and respiratory muscles, along with loss of reflexes, at which time the diagnosis becomes obvious.

Axonal GBS

In 1986, Dr. Thomas Feasby and his associates in Canada published a description of five people with GBS who had prominent damage of axons rather than of the myelin sheaths. They called this *axonal GBS.* Tissue specimens from one person documented the axonal damage as the cause of paralysis. All five patients had rapidly progressive paralysis of four limbs and loss of reflexes. Three patients required breathing support within a day or two of the onset of symptoms. Three patients had experienced recent diarrhea, and one had had an upper respiratory infection. In all five patients, weakness progressed so rapidly that they sought medical care and were admitted to a hospital from less than 24 hours to 2 days after the onset of their first symptoms. Four patients had major alterations of internal organ (autonomic) nerve supply, with major swings in blood pressure or heart rate. All developed muscle atrophy or wasting. The prognosis, or outcome, of this form of GBS is poor. One patient died and of the four who survived, one required mechanical ventilation for 11 months and still could not stand or walk by 16 months. After 1 year, the other three patients could walk with leg braces or a cane. In all five of them, electrical stimulation of the nerve supply to most of their major limb muscles did not produce any response. The authors mentioned two additional cases with similar severe symptoms; nerve biopsies in both cases showed extensive axonal damage without myelin involvement.

Since the Feasby publication, others have reported similar cases in which there was biopsy-proven axonal damage without myelin involvement. Axonal GBS is now accepted as a variant of classic GBS, and has been given a longer descriptive name and accompanying abbreviation, as discussed in Chapter 1.

Axonal GBS makes up approximately 10 percent of the cases of GBS in Western countries. A diagnosis of axonal GBS is supported by the rapid onset of paralysis, with inexcitable motor nerves on electrophysiologic testing and a poor outcome. It is treated in the same way as classic (demyelinating) GBS: with IVIG or plasma exchange and supportive care.

THE EVOLUTION FROM WEAKNESS TO IMPROVEMENT

GBS is a disease that evolves rapidly. There may be a few days of vague numbness or tingling prior to the development of weakness. Approximately 50 percent of cases reach maximum weakness within about a week. Ninety percent of cases reach this point by 3 weeks, and progression stops by 4 weeks by definition. Then, there is a plateau phase during which time neither deterioration nor improvement occurs. Recovery of strength typically begins 2 to 4 weeks after maximum weakness is reached. It may begin without an obvious plateau of weakness in mild cases. The patient may remain quite weak for several months in severe cases. Severity of weakness and the rate and degree of recovery vary enormously. Not surprisingly, the more severely the individual is affected, the slower and less complete his or her recovery. In mild cases, complete recovery may occur over a few weeks, while other cases can take years. In severe cases, the majority of recovery occurs within 1 to 2 years, although continued slow improvement occurs over much longer periods.

GBS develops rapidly and progresses for up to 4 weeks. Then, there is a brief plateau, followed by steady improvement over subsequent months. Strength is fully recovered in approximately 75 percent of cases, although other residual effects may persist permanently.

Relapses in true GBS are rare, occurring in perhaps 2 to 5 percent of cases. Progressive improvement is the norm once a person begins to recover. Occasionally, people with CIDP are initially diagnosed with GBS, but then relapse weeks or months later, at which time the correct diagnosis can be made.

The prognosis in GBS is generally good. In approximately 70 to 80 percent of cases there is a complete return of strength. About 5 percent of cases are fatal, and the rest are left with variable degrees of weakness. It is becoming increasingly evident that minor but extremely annoying symptoms may persist for years, sometimes permanently, as will be discussed further in a later section.

INVOLVEMENT OF THE CENTRAL NERVOUS SYSTEM

As discussed in Chapter 1, GBS is a disorder affecting peripheral nerves—the nerves that go from the brain to the limbs, internal organs, and muscles involved in respiration. However, some people have involvement of the CNS (the brain and spinal cord). This involvement is invariably mild and has little clinical consequence. It is often restricted to mild abnormalities on a magnetic resonance imaging (MRI) scan. It is important to recognize that CNS involvement may occur so that diagnostic confusion can be avoided. The finding of MRI abnormalities or other signs of CNS involvement should certainly raise questions about the diagnosis, but it should not result in withholding prompt treatment in an otherwise typical case. Probably the most common clinically significant abnormality of the CNS is involvement of the optic nerve, which causes blurred vision in one eye. Occasionally, there may be evidence of mild transverse myelitis associated with true GBS. A much more common cause of CNS involvement in people with GBS is a secondary effect from medications, or from lack of oxygen due to breathing failure, causing confusion and excessive sleepiness.

The central nervous system may occasionally be involved in GBS, but this is seldom clinically significant. Minimal involvement of the brain and spinal cord should not distract the neurologist from the correct diagnosis in an otherwise typical case of GBS.

CHAPTER 3

How Is Guillain-Barré Syndrome Diagnosed?

The diagnosis Guillain-Barre syndrome (GBS) is based on the characteristic clinical features of acutely evolving weakness and loss of reflexes following an antecedent illness, such as an upper respiratory tract infection or diarrhea. However, because of the conditions that can mimic GBS, as discussed in Chapter 2, confirmation of the diagnosis by way of various diagnostic tests adds to the confidence of a correct diagnosis. The most commonly used diagnostic tests are electrophysiologic studies and examination of the cerebrospinal fluid (CSF), which is obtained by spinal tap *(lumbar puncture).* The results of these tests usually provide positive confirmation of the clinical suspicion. If the diagnosis remains in doubt, other tests may be necessary to ensure that some other disease is not masquerading as GBS.

ELECTRODIAGNOSTIC TESTING IN GUILLAIN-BARRÉ SNYDROME

Electrodiagnostic testing of nerves and muscles is an integral part of diagnosing GBS and its variants.

In addition, the tests can provide an estimate of prognosis.

WHY DO ELECTRODIAGNOSTIC TESTING?

A diagnosis of GBS is usually suspected based on the clinical presentation. The combination of the history and the physical findings is often enough for the doctor to make a working diagnosis of GBS. However, a definitive diagnosis is important for proper treatment and prognosis and to plan treatment. Given the risk of respiratory failure and the ability to hasten recovery with appropriate immune-modulating therapies, it is imperative to quickly establish the correct diagnosis so that treatment can be instituted in a timely fashion and in an appropriate setting. Obviously, a person with tick paralysis, arsenic poisoning, or some other disorder that mimics GBS should not be treated as if they had GBS. Conversely, the doctor would not want to manage a person who is deteriorating with GBS anywhere other than in the intensive care unit (ICU).

Electrical testing of nerve function can be done in almost any setting, including the emergency room and the ICU, but it is usually done in a specialized laboratory. Results are available as soon as the test is completed. The electromyographic (EMG) and nerve conduction study results can establish that GBS is the correct diagnosis, and they can exclude other causes of acutely evolving weakness. While the testing may be painful, it is safe and relatively noninvasive. Therefore, electrical testing is the appropriate next step in the diagnostic evaluation of a person suspected of having GBS.

Before describing electrical testing, it will be helpful to first provide some basic information about the structure (anatomy) and function (physiology) of peripheral nerves.

ANATOMY OF A NERVE

Figure 3-1a shows a normally myelinated motor nerve. The main part of the cell, the cell body, lies in the spinal cord or in the brain stem of cranial nerves. The axon extends from the cell body to the muscle, which may be located in an arm, leg, or elsewhere. The normal axon is myelinated—meaning it is covered with an insulating layer of myelin to prevent leakage of the electrical current that flows down the axon from the cell body to the muscle. The myelin sheath is not a continuous structure, but is made up of segments of myelin separated by tiny gaps (nodes of Ranvier). These gaps are where the current flowing along the nerve is regenerated.

Figure 3-1b depicts what happens in people with the demyelinating form of GBS. Some of the segments of myelin degenerate and are stripped away from the underlying axon, removing the insulation and leading to a "short circuit." The axon remains intact, but the current leaks out and the message fails to reach the muscle, resulting in weakness.

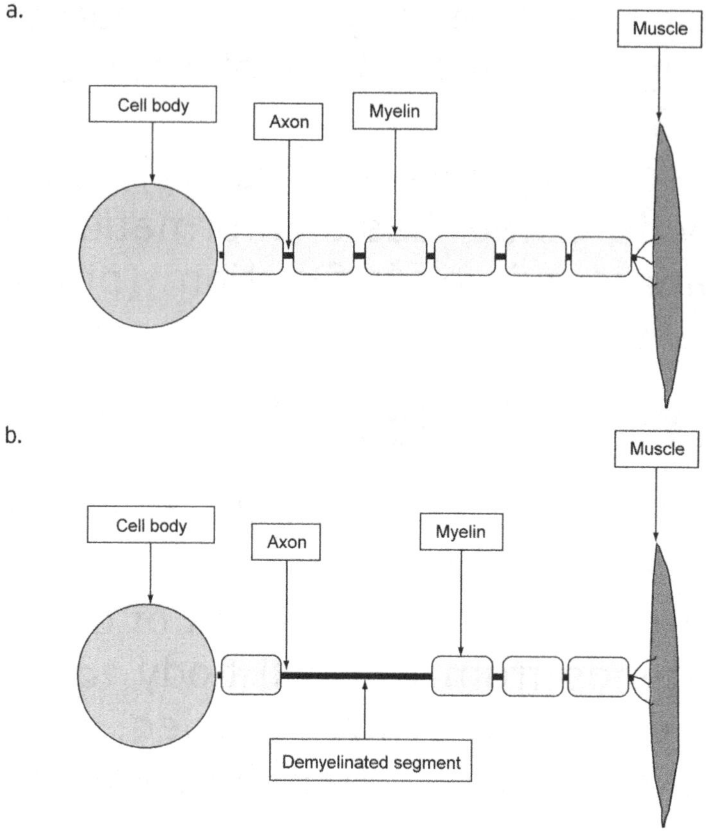

FIGURES 3-1a and b: (a). Schematic representation of a normal motor unit. The nerve cell body and the motor neuron lie in the spinal cord. The axon extends all the way from the spinal cord to the muscle, which may be located anywhere in the limbs. After it enters the muscle, the motor axon divides into many tiny branches, each of which provides a nerve supply to a single muscle fiber. Thus, each motor neuron provides a nerve supply to many muscle fibers. The myelin sheath is a discontinuous structure consisting of segments of myelin insulation with tiny gaps called the nodes of Ranvier, where the electrical current is generated and renewed. (b). In GBS, the myelin sheath is damaged and removed (demyelination), leaving a segment of non-insulated axon that cannot conduct electrical impulses. This leads to muscle weakness. In reality, the demyelination is a patchy process occurring at multiple sites along the length of the axon, most prominently at a point closest to the cell body.

c.

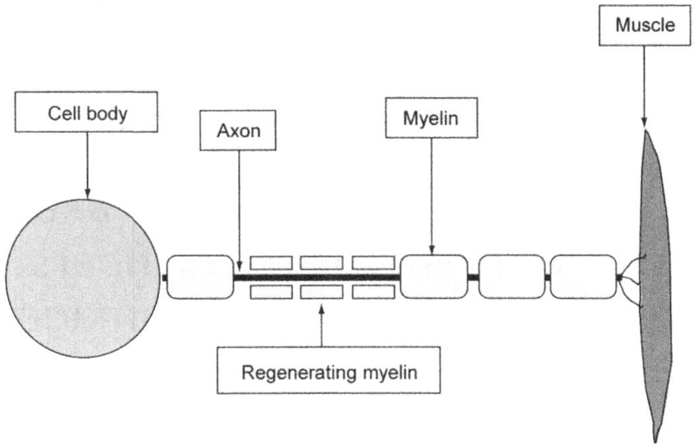

FIGURE 3-1c: After the myelin debris is removed, new myelin is formed, restoring the insulating sheath and allowing electrical conduction to be restored.

The myelin then regenerates and reconstitutes the insulating layer, as shown in Figure 3-1c. Initially, the newly formed myelin is thinner and the segments are shorter. The myelin becomes thicker and forms a more effective insulating layer over time. Conduction of electrical impulses in the underlying axon becomes normal, or nearly normal.

Damage in GBS often starts in the most proximal part of the nerve (the nerve root), as it emerges from the spinal cord. Damage is most prominent in the motor *nerve root,* which lies *anteriorly* (in the front). The sensory nerve root emerges from the back part of the spinal cord. The motor and sensory nerve roots fuse to form the spinal nerve that emerges from the bony canal of the spine, which is then joined by the autonomic nerve fibers. The nerve containing motor, sensory, and autonomic fibers then travels out into the body and limbs, where the fibers join the muscles, skin, and vital organs. At the far, or distal, end of the motor nerves, where they enter the muscle, each motor nerve fiber (axon) divides into many small branches, which go to individual muscle fibers. Thus, each motor axon provides a nerve supply to many muscle fibers. These end branches are also where myelin damage tends to occur relatively early in GBS. Each nerve contains thousands of individual motor, sensory, and autonomic axons.

FUNCTIONS OF NERVES

The nerves of the human body function in much the same way as electrical wires in a house.

The nerves of the human body function in much the same way as electrical wires in a house.

The axon is equivalent to the copper wire that carries electrical impulses, and the myelin provides insulation so that the current is not lost through a short circuit. The amount of electrical activity in human nerves is very small, but extremely sensitive instruments have been devised to measure it. Abnormal patterns of electrical activity are recognized that closely reflect the underlying damage to the nerve.

Thus, the type of injury to the nerve can be inferred from the electrical studies without having to remove the nerve from the body for microscopic examination.

Electrical testing of nerves and muscles is often known collectively as *electromyography* (EMG), but there are actually two separate components of the test. Nerve conduction studies are the most important part of the electrophysiologic testing in GBS. The term *electromyography* should really be reserved for that part of the test where a needle is inserted into the muscle.

NERVE CONDUCTION STUDIES

The nerve conduction study (NCS) is the most important part of electrodiagnostic testing in people with GBS. In this test, electrical shocks are administered through the skin to activate the nerves. The shock is administered at several different sites along the course of the nerve, usually at least two sites, but sometimes more. Shocks are given using a small, hand-held device, as shown in Figure 3-2. The responses can be recorded with small discs that stick to the skin or, less commonly, with small needles inserted just under the skin. These electrical shocks are uncomfortable, but they do not cause any harm because the amount of current extremely is small. There is no risk of burning the skin or damaging the nerves. The electrical impulse travels along the nerve, and can be recorded from the muscle that it supplies *(motor NCS)* or directly from sensory nerve fiber bundles *(sensory NCS).*

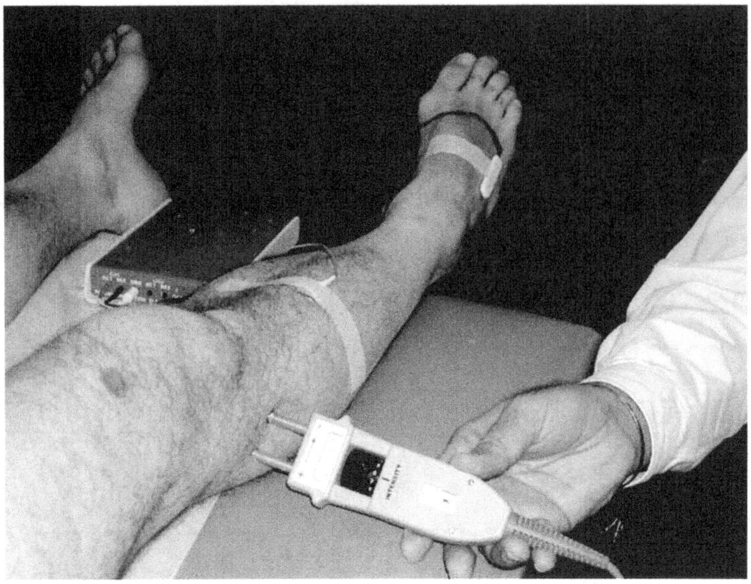

FIGURE 3-2: Motor nerve conduction studies being done in the peroneal nerve, one of the leg nerves. The electrodes that record responses are attached to the top of the foot and lie over the muscle that is being activated. The handheld stimulator is applied to the peroneal nerve near the knee. The nerve can also be activated by stimulation at the ankle. In this way, the time that it takes for the electrical impulse to travel from each site of stimulation (knee and ankle) can be measured by the instrument, and the speed of conduction can be calculated for the distance between the knee and the ankle.

An example of the motor nerve conduction studies from a normal individual and from a person with GBS is shown in Figure 3-3. The size of the electrical response and the time it takes for the impulse to travel from the site of stimulation to the recording site can be measured. The speed of conduction can then be calculated. The size of the response reflects the number of functioning nerves connected to muscle fibers. The speed of conduction reflects the integrity of the myelin sheath. Electrical impulses in normal human peripheral nerves travel at 40 to 45 meters per second (m/sec) in the legs and 50 to 65 m/sec in the arms. In classic GBS, in which the myelin sheath is damaged, the conduction speed is severely slowed, sometimes below 20 m/sec, but the size of the response is normal or nearly normal because most of the axons remain intact. In axonal GBS, the conduction speed is normal, but the size of the response is very small because the axons have degenerated. The prognosis for full recovery of strength is poor if the size of the electrical response is less than 10 percent of normal. Abnormalities of nerve conduction appear very soon after the onset of GBS; some changes may be seen within the first day. However, nerve conduction study results can become progressively more abnormal over a period of several weeks, and can continue to worsen—even as the person with GBS begins to improve.

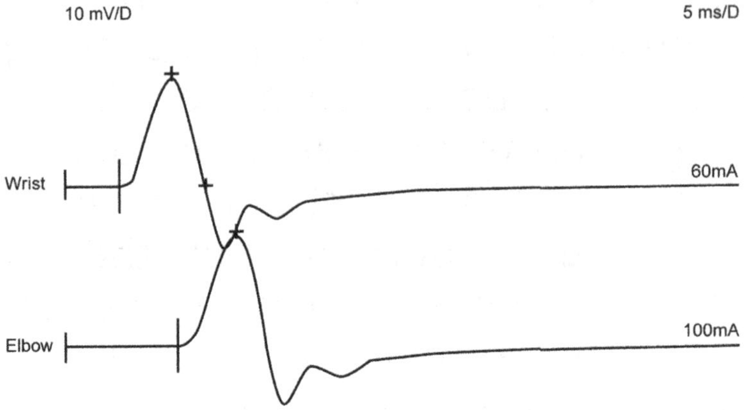

dLAT/CV	AMP	AREA	DUR
4.2	10.3	34.7	6.5
61.6 m/s	−1%	0%	3%
8.5	10.2	34.8	6.7

FIGURE 3-3a: (a). Motor nerve conduction studies recorded from one of the arm nerves, the median nerve, in a normal individual. The amplitude of the responses (the height to the peak of each tracing) is a little more than 10 millivolts (mV), and is about the same whether the nerve is stimulated at the wrist or the elbow (the second column of figures), which is normal. The time it takes for the impulse to travel from the wrist to the muscle is 4.2 m/sec. From the elbow to the muscle is 8.5 msec, and the speed of conduction from the elbow to the wrist is 61.6 meters per second (m/s) (the first column of figures).

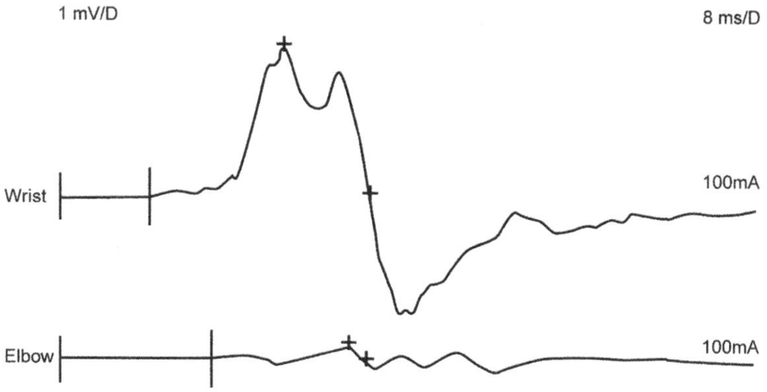

dLAT/CV	AMP	AREA	DUR
10.7	1.4	13.4	24.7
40.6 m/s	–92%	–96%	–30%
17.6	0.1	0.5	17.3

FIGURE 3-3b: (b). Motor nerve conduction studies recorded from the median nerve in a 37-year-old man with GBS who has been weak for 8 days. The amplitude of the response when the nerve is stimulated at the wrist is 1.4 mV. The amplitude with stimulation at the elbow is only 0.1 mV. These are both abnormal responses, but they are more than 10 percent of normal, indicating a good prognosis for recovery. The time it takes for the impulse to travel from the wrist to the muscle is severely prolonged at 10.7 msec, and the speed of conduction between wrist and elbow is very slow at 40.6 m/sec.

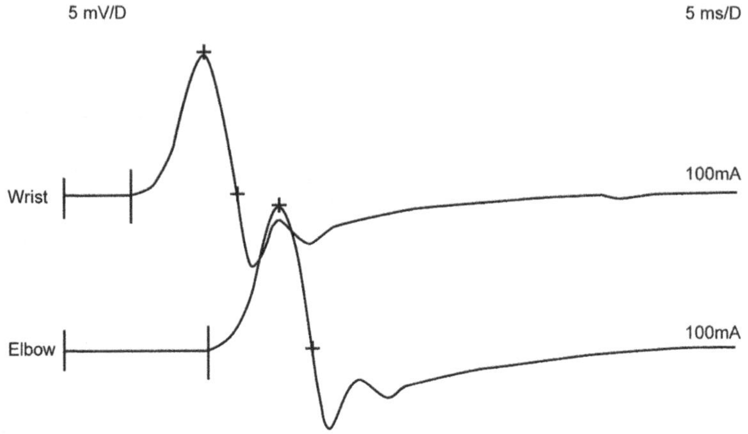

dLAT/CV	AMP	AREA	DUR
5.4	6.6	24.4	7.8
45.6 m/s	1%	–1%	–2%
11.1	6.7	24.2	7.7

FIGURE 3-3c: (c). Motor nerve conduction studies in the median nerve in the same patient as Fig. 3-3(b) recorded 5 months later. The amplitudes are now normal and the speed of conduction has improved, but it is not quite back to normal. The patient has now completely recovered his strength and motor function.

ELECTROMYOGRAPHY (EMG)

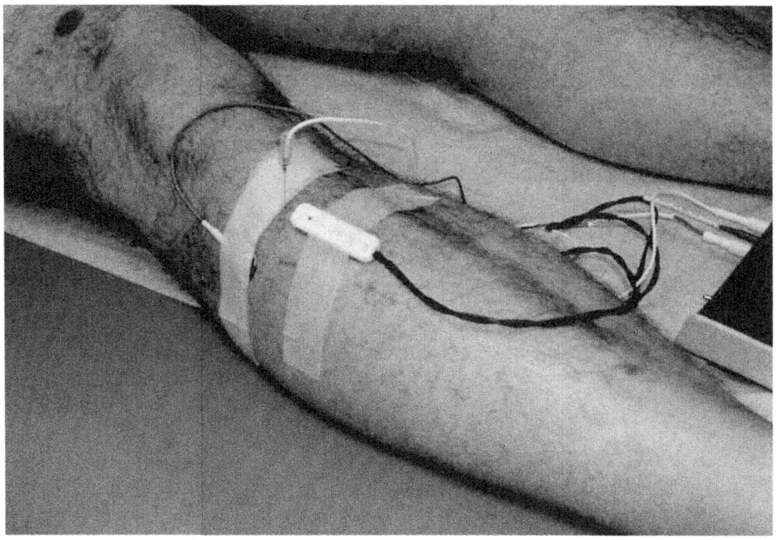

FIGURE 3-4: Needle electromyography (EMG). In the EMG portion of the test, a fine needle is inserted into the muscle to record the electrical activity, both with the muscle fully relaxed and during voluntary muscle contraction.

EMG plays a negligible role in the diagnosis of GBS, but it is an important supplementary tool to assess the degree of axonal damage. The electromyogram provides critical information regarding prognosis. As shown in Figure 3-4, during this test, a small needle is inserted into the muscle. This needle senses the electrical activity of the muscle. The EMG machine then transforms this activity into a visual and an *aural* (audible) signal. Initially, the needle is inserted with the muscle completely relaxed. It is then moved quickly through the muscle so that several different areas can be sampled. No electrical activity should be present in a normal, relaxed muscle. The person being tested is then asked to gently contract the muscle, so that the muscle fibers are activated and the electrical activity of those muscle fibers can be recorded and analyzed.

There will be abnormal electrical activity in the relaxed muscle when there has been damage to the nerve fibers that supply that muscle. This abnormal electrical activity is called *fibrillation.* This activity does not appear immediately after the onset of GBS, and will not show on an electromyogram performed early. This is why the people suspected of having GBS are often asked to return to the EMG laboratory for a second study a few weeks after the initial study. Some research studies have shown that the prognosis of GBS is related to the degree of fibrillation—in other words, the more fibrillation, the less of a recovery, but this is not a consistent finding. The pattern of activation recorded during gentle voluntary contraction of the muscle can provide further information regarding the severity of degeneration of the axons.

There are a few caveats about studying people with suspected GBS. Early in the disorder, only some nerves may have sufficient damage to be detected with electrical testing. Therefore, when GBS is suspected, it is prudent to study multiple nerves, especially in areas that are clinically abnormal, so as to not miss abnormalities that will help confirm the suspected diagnosis. If only one nerve is studied and found to have only one abnormality, one might be suspicious of GBS, but still be skeptical without finding other

NCV abnormalities typical of GBS in that nerve or in other nerves. It is therefore prudent to study other nerves and nerves in other limbs to look for additional abnormalities, such as slowed conduction velocity or prolonged distal latencies, which indicate widespread demyelination that more strongly supports a diagnosis of GBS. The most important diagnostic feature of the electrophysiologic studies is demonstration of the characteristic evolution of the changes, not necessarily the static changes seen during one study. Thus, if the diagnosis is uncertain, the studies may need to be repeated.

In conclusion, the presence, location, and type of nerve damage can be identified via nerve conduction studies and EMG in order to verify the diagnosis of GBS.

CEREBROSPINAL FLUID (CSF) TESTING IN GUILLAIN-BARRÉ SYNDROME

The lumbar puncture is a technique whereby a fine needle is inserted into the lower back under local anesthetic, and a few teaspoons of the fluid that bathes the brain and spinal cord are withdrawn. There is widespread anxiety about this procedure, but it is usually simple and safe. It does entail insertion of a needle, and it is therefore uncomfortable. Also, about 25 percent of the people who undergo this procedure experience some headache after the fluid is removed, but it is severe only about 5 percent of cases. The procedure is difficult to perform and may need to be done under x-ray guidance if the person is extremely obese or has had previous back surgery.

The characteristic abnormality of the CSF in GBS is an increased protein concentration with normal numbers of cells, which is the albuminocytologic dissociation, described nearly 100 years ago by Guillain, Barré, and Strohl. Normally, the CSF contains 15 to 60 milligrams of protein for every 100 milliliters of fluid (expressed as mg/dl). This is elevated in the majority of people with GBS. The protein concentration is usually above 100 mg/dl, and it may be very high indeed, occasionally over 1,000 mg/dl. Once the protein level is above 150 mg/dl, the CSF, which is normally crystal clear, becomes faintly yellow. The protein may be normal in the very earliest stages of the disease, but it is nearly always elevated by the end of the first week. If the protein is normal at the time of the first spinal tap, it may be necessary to repeat the test a week or so later if the diagnosis remains in doubt. Normal CSF contains a few white blood cells (lymphocytes); usually no more than five cells per milliliter of fluid. Early reports of GBS emphasized the absence of cells, and that is often the case. In other words, the cell count is not increased above normal. However, a small increase in the numbers of lymphocytes may be seen, particularly early in the course of the disease. The diagnostic criteria that were developed through the National Institutes of Health allow for as many as 50 cells/ml of CSF. A second spinal tap will probably be recommended if the lymphocyte cell count in the CSF is above 20 cells/ml. GBS is often associated with viral infections, which may cause inflammation of the *meninges* that line the brain and spinal cord, leading to inflammatory cells spilling into the CSF. It is therefore not surprising that a few lymphocytes can be seen in the early stages of GBS. People with *human immunodeficiency virus* (HIV) infection may also get GBS. In these cases, lymphocyte counts up to 50 cells/ml may be seen. If the lymphocyte count is above 50 cells/ml, other diseases, including poliomyelitis, West Nile fever, or some other viral infection, should be seriously considered. Inflammatory cells other than lymphocytes should not be seen in the CSF of people with GBS and, if present, this should raise serious concerns about the diagnosis of GBS and other diagnoses need to be considered. The concentration of *glucose* (sugar) in normal CSF is 40 to 80 mg/dl. This is not altered in people with GBS.

OTHER LABORATORY TESTING

There are no blood tests that can provide assistance in establishing a diagnosis of GBS. Specifically, the white blood cell count is usually normal, and no antibodies against nerve components can be reliably detected in the blood. Blood testing is done to exclude other conditions or to establish the nature of any antecedent infection that has led to GBS. Antibodies to the microorganisms that trigger GBS *can* be detected.

The common triggering agents that can be identified in this fashion include *cytomegalovirus* (CMV), *Epstein-Barr virus* (EBV, the virus that causes infectious *mononucleosis),* and the bacterium *Campylobacter jejuni,* one of the most common causes of food poisoning.

People with GBS may occasionally develop a low serum sodium concentration that can lead to confusion, drowsiness, and occasionally seizures, so careful monitoring of the electrolytes in the blood is important during the early days of illness.

People with GBS often have x-ray studies or *magnetic resonance imaging* (MRI) scans. These tests are not typically necessary, but they may be useful if there are unusual features that make the diagnosis uncertain. For example, as discussed in Chapter 2, inflammation of the spinal cord (transverse myelitis) may mimic GBS. An MRI of the spine is indicated if this is suspected. Usually, an MRI of the brain will be done if there is prominent involvement of cranial nerves. For example, people with Miller Fisher syndrome often have an MRI scan of their brain.

Nerve biopsy, to allow for examination of a piece of nerve under the microscope, is often done to assist in the diagnosis of the related disorder CIDP, but this test is rarely indicated in GBS.

CHAPTER 4

What Causes Guillain-Barré Syndrome?

INCIDENCE OF GUILLAIN-BARRÉ SNYDROME

The incidence of any disease is the frequency with which it occurs in a defined population over a specific period of time. Traditionally, this is described as an "annual incidence," meaning the number of cases that occur in a year. GBS is a rare disease. In North America, there are approximately 1.5 to 2.0 cases of GBS for every 100,000 people each year. This means there are about 4,000 to 4,500 new cases each year in the United States. Occasionally, there are apparent outbreaks of GBS. For example, there was a increase in the number of cases that occurred following the U.S. swine influenza vaccination program in 1976. Another such outbreak, although a much smaller one, occurred in one county in Colorado in 1981, when the incidence was 4.0/100,000. During the preceding 5 years, the incidence had been 1.2/100,000. Surrounding counties did not experience the same increase. No explanation for this outbreak has ever been found. Other short-lived outbreaks have been described from around the world, usually following epidemics of infectious illnesses, but sometimes with no apparent cause.

GBS is a rare disease that affects people from all parts of the world. It is a little more common in men, occurs in all age groups, and is rare in children.

GBS affects males and females of all ages and races. It is rare in children, particularly during the first 2 years of life, and tends to increase in frequency throughout life, although there is a small peak in frequency in young adults. In most surveys, the incidence is only slightly higher for men and in Caucasians, although one Minnesota study showed that men outnumbered women by almost 2:1. One curious feature is the lack of a particular seasonal preponderance, at least in Western countries. Given the relationship of GBS to colds and flu-like illnesses, it is expected that GBS would occur more frequently in the fall and winter when these infections are more likely.

TRIGGERING EVENTS

GBS is an autoimmune disease that affects peripheral nerves. The normal function of the immune system is to recognize and eliminate invaders from outside the body, such as bacteria and viruses, and to eliminate damaged cells within the body, such as cancer cells. In autoimmune diseases, for reasons that are unclear, this response is misdirected, and the immune system turns against the body, causing disease. There are many different types of autoimmune disease, and they affect almost any organ of the body, including rheumatoid arthritis, ulcerative colitis, juvenile (insulin-dependent) diabetes, systemic *lupus erythematosus* (lupus), multiple sclerosis, and many others. The immune attack in GBS is directed against peripheral nerves, most often the myelin sheath. In some cases, autoimmune diseases are triggered by a recognized antecedent event, presumably an event that nonspecifically stimulates the immune system. In GBS, about two-thirds to three-quarters of the people affected are able to identify an illness or event that occurred a week or two prior to the development of weakness. Most commonly, this illness is an infection. GBS can also occur after some vaccinations and following surgery or other trauma. Regardless of the triggering event, the neurologic symptoms appear an average of 2 weeks after the triggering event, although they may appear as early as 1 week and as late as 4 weeks. One consistent observation is that the shorter the interval between the antecedent event and the onset of neurologic symptoms, the more severe the GBS.

GBS is an autoimmune disease in which the immune attack is directed against peripheral nerves.

> Most people with GBS are able to identify an event that triggered the attack.

Guillain-Barré Syndrome Following Infections

Many different kinds of infections can trigger an attack of GBS—most commonly a respiratory infection that causes cold or influenza-like symptoms, such as fever, runny nose, cough, and generalized aches and pains. There is no relationship between the severity of symptoms and the subsequent development of GBS; a person is just as likely to get GBS following a minor flu-like episode as following a severe episode. In the majority of cases, the specific infectious organism is never identified, partly because the infection has subsided by the time GBS appears, and partly, because most doctors do not bother to look for it. *Cytomegalovirus* and an unusual bacterium called *Mycoplasma pneumoniae* are examples of microorganisms that cause respiratory illness and can then trigger GBS. The second most common antecedent illness is gastroenteritis, which causes diarrhea and sometimes nausea and vomiting. Again, the exact identity of the infecting organism is usually unknown, but when carefully sought, infection with *Campylobacter jejuni,* a common food contaminant, is the most frequently identified culprit. The virus that causes infectious mononucleosis (Epstein Barr virus, or EBV) can also be a trigger. GBS is also associated with HIV, the virus that causes AIDS. It usually occurs in the early stages of HIV, before the immune system is severely compromised; perhaps shortly after the initial infection. GBS has been reported following an extremely wide range of other viral and bacterial infections, but those discussed above seem to have a particular propensity to trigger the disease. One of the older names for GBS was *acute infectious polyneuritis,* implying that it was an infection of the nerves. However, GBS is caused by the immune system reacting to an infection. There is no actual infection of the nerves.

The most common trigger for GBS is infection, usually a flu-like illness or diarrhea. In most cases, the specific infectious organism is not identified. The virus or bacterium that triggers GBS does not actually infect the nerve.

Guillain-Barré Syndrome Following Vaccination

GBS can also follow certain types of vaccination. The best-known example is the association of GBS with the U.S. swine influenza vaccination program of 1976. In the fall of that year, approximately 50 million people in the United States were vaccinated with a vaccine containing *A/New Jersey swine influenza virus* in a program sponsored by the federal government. There was an increase in the frequency of GBS in the people who received the vaccine during the months that followed. Between October 1, 1976, and January 31, 1977, there were 1,098 cases reported to the Centers for Disease Control and Prevention (CDC). Of these, 532 had received the vaccine prior to the onset of GBS. This represented a more than 20-fold increase in the number of cases expected to occur in nonvaccinated individuals. Prior to that time, only three cases of GBS associated with influenza vaccine had been reported despite the widespread incorporation of swine influenza virus into vaccines administered to military personnel in the 1950s and 1960s. Furthermore, a subsequent vaccination program between 1978 and 1979, using a vaccine that did not contain swine influenza virus, caused no increase in the expected incidence of GBS. Thus, the 1976 outbreak appears to have been specific for this particular vaccine.

GBS may possibly occur following vaccination for polio. During 1985, following an outbreak of polio in Finland, 94 percent of the population was vaccinated over a 5-week period. In one district in southern Finland, there was a marked increase in the number of GBS cases seen over the next 4 months. There have been no other reports of GBS following polio vaccination.

The first reports of GBS following vaccination appeared in the nineteenth century. Shortly after the introduction of rabies vaccination by Pasteur in the late 1890s, there were neurologic complications, including acute polyneuritis. This complication was related to contamination of the vaccine with nerve tissue, but it has virtually disappeared in those areas of the world where the vaccine is prepared from duck or chick embryos. However, vaccine is still prepared from nerve tissue in developing countries, and GBS following rabies vaccination continues to occasionally occur in those parts of the world. When it does occur following rabies vaccination, GBS has a high incidence of severe cranial nerve involvement, and is unusually severe with a high mortality rate.

Recently, there have been reports of GBS after vaccination against the *meningococcal bacterium,* which causes a form of meningitis. In 2005, five people developed GBS a few weeks after receiving the vaccine. It is not known exactly how many people received this particular vaccine, and therefore it is impossible to determine whether this represents a significantly increased risk. However, the cases occurred 2 to 4 weeks after receiving the vaccine, strongly suggesting that the vaccine was the trigger. More research is needed before deciding whether the risk of getting GBS following this type of vaccination outweighs the risk of getting meningitis.

Vaccination rarely triggers GBS. The swine influenza vaccination program of 1976 caused an increase in the number of cases of GBS. No other vaccine has been consistently associated with GBS.

The association between GBS and other types of vaccination has not been established. While there appear to be individuals who develop GBS after being vaccinated, there does not appear to be an increased risk for the general population; nor is there any risk that people who have had GBS will relapse if they are vaccinated.

Guillain-Barré Syndrome Following Surgery

About 5 percent of GBS cases are said to follow surgery, although this is controversial. GBS has been described following surgery to the head, chest, abdomen, and limbs. In some cases, the surgery has been complicated by infection; in others, the surgery has been uncomplicated. Cases have been described using either spinal or general anesthesia. It has been suggested that in GBS following surgery there tends to be a short interval between the surgery and the onset of neurologic symptoms. GBS arising after surgery may be particularly severe.

Guillain-Barré Syndrome Associated with Pregnancy

By the year 2001, published reports indicated that at least 50 cases of GBS during pregnancy had been documented. GBS during pregnancy can start in any trimester or shortly after delivery of the baby. There is no evidence that pregnancy or delivery increases the risk of developing GBS; nor is there evidence to suggest that pregnancy adversely affects the outcome of GBS. The effects on pregnancy from the treatment of GBS are usually minimal. Supportive care is the same for both pregnant and nonpregnant women with GBS. For example, if sufficient breathing difficulties develop, mechanical ventilation can be used without increased harm to the mother or fetus. Both plasma exchange and, to a lesser extent, intravenous immunoglobulin (IVIg) therapy have been used during all three trimesters without adverse problems to either mother or fetus. The risk of using immune globulin in pregnancy is defined as category C, indicating lack of evidence of any harm to the fetus. If a woman has had GBS during pregnancy, there is no evidence of increased risk of recurrence during subsequent pregnancies.

A close relationship between the neurologist treating the GBS and the obstetrician managing the pregnancy is important when GBS develops during pregnancy. In addition to plasma exchange and IVIg, people with GBS *often* need other treatments, such as anticoagulants (blood thinners) to prevent blood clots and antibiotics if infections develop. The anticoagulant warfarin (Coumadin®) has been associated with an increased incidence of fetal abnormalities, and it should not be used during the first trimester of pregnancy unless the health of the mother requires it. Heparin can be given by daily injection, and it is probably a safer alternative to use as an anticoagulant. Most antibiotics are safe, but consultation with a pharmacist may be wise before using any drug during the first trimester of pregnancy when the risk of developmental abnormalities is at its highest. In addition, if a woman who is recovering from GBS is on warfarin or any other drug, it is advisable to delay pregnancy until she is no longer on medication.

Healthy Babies Borne of Women with GBS

Mothers with GBS can deliver their babies both vaginally and by cesarean section, and the babies are just as likely to be healthy as infants born of a mother who does not have GBS. The decision as to method of delivery depends on the standard obstetric assessment. The first and second stages of labor can proceed normally in the pregnant woman with GBS, but the third stage, when the mother is asked to push to help deliver the baby, may be more difficult. Theoretically, this stage could also lead to more autonomic abnormalities, but this has not been specifically reported. GBS does not affect fetal development or infant health. Specifically, there is no evidence of an increased risk of congenital abnormalities, and there is no need to consider terminating a pregnancy because of the GBS.

Third Trimester GBS

Development of severe GBS in the third trimester is associated with an increased risk of aspiration pneumonia in the mother. The likelihood of premature birth is increased in severe, third trimester GBS. Labor and delivery can proceed if the mother is on a ventilator.

GBS in an Infant

There is only one reported case of maternal GBS followed by development of GBS in the infant. A woman who developed GBS at week 29 (the beginning of the third trimester) delivered a healthy boy vaginally at 38 weeks while she was improving but still on a ventilator. Blood tests showed she had experienced a recent viral infection (cytomegalovirus). At 12 days of age, the baby developed findings of GBS, with poor and then absent reflexes, widespread muscle weakness, and breathing difficulties leading to mechanical ventilation. He had elevated spinal fluid protein as well as electrophysiologic evidence of GBS. The baby received high-dose intravenous IVIg therapy with good response, and had a normal examination by day 14. This is the youngest reported case of GBS, and also the first report of the use of IVIg for neonatal GBS.

Women can develop GBS during pregnancy, but this is coincidental. Pregnancy does not affect the severity of GBS, and GBS does not affect the outcome of the pregnancy or the fetus. Treatment during pregnancy is no different than treatment of nonpregnant women, and there is no increased risk of developing GBS in subsequent pregnancies.

WHY DO INFECTIONS AND OTHER EVENTS TRIGGER GULLAIN-BARRÉ SYNDROME?

The answer to this question is partly conjectural, but it is also partly based on sound scientific evidence. The most well-established mechanism is a phenomenon called *molecular mimicry.* The immune system is designed so that it can recognize certain molecules on the surface of infecting organisms and identify them as foreign invaders. These molecules are called *antigens.* Once an antigen has been identified as belonging to an invader, the immune system, through an extremely complex cascade of events, develops antibodies against the antigen and recruits inflammatory cells that destroy the invading organism. These antibodies may attack an organ of the host if the molecular structure of the antigen is sufficiently similar to an antigen of the host. In the case of GBS, if the antigen of the invading organism is similar to the antigens on the surface of the myelin sheath, then antibodies and inflammatory cells will attack and damage the myelin. In this case, a molecule on the surface of the invader "mimics" a molecule in the body of the infected individual. There are some organisms that have such a strong similarity to human myelin molecules that they are particularly likely to induce an attack of GBS. This is best demonstrated by the bacterium *Campylobacter jejuni,* which has molecules on its surface that seem to be particularly likely to induce GBS. This may also be the case with the viruses CMV and EBV because they are also common triggers for GBS, although molecular mimicry has not been proven for these two viruses.

If this phenomenon is the basis for all cases of GBS, then it is possible that any antecedent infection or vaccination has a small possibility of triggering GBS in a susceptible individual if there is sufficient similarity between the unique molecular structure of that individual's myelin and the molecular structure of the invader. However, there may be a small number of organisms that more frequently resemble the molecular structure of human myelin, and therefore have a high likelihood triggering an attack of GBS. This may explain why the 1976 swine influenza vaccination program triggered so many cases of GBS. Perhaps the molecular structure of that particular vaccine had a high molecular similarity to human myelin. Other vaccines trigger GBS in certain susceptible individuals even though they do *not* have sufficient similarity to the molecular structure of the myelin in most individuals. This would explain the occasional person who has an attack of GBS following an influenza vaccination without an overall increase in the number of cases of GBS.

Infections are thought to trigger GBS by the mechanism of molecular mimicry, whereby the infecting organism sufficiently resembles peripheral nerve antigens and the immune system reacts to the infection and attacks the nerve.

What Happens to the Nerves in GBS?

As discussed in previous chapters, peripheral nerves consist of an electrical cable (axon) and an insulating sheath (myelin). The axon is responsible for transmitting signals between the brain and the rest of the body. The sensory axons transmit messages from the periphery of the body to the brain; the motor axons transmit messages from the brain to the muscles. The insulating properties of the myelin prevent leakage of electrical current (a short circuit), which helps to ensure the efficient functioning of the peripheral nervous system.

Myelin is formed by a specific cell in the peripheral nerve called the *Schwann cell* so-named for the scientist who first described the cell. In the most common form of GBS, the demyelinating form, the immune system attacks the myelin, as described above. The damaged myelin degenerates and is engulfed by cells that function as scavengers, the *macrophages.* When the affected nerves of people with GBS are examined under the microscope, the first abnormality to be seen is the migration of inflammatory cells and macrophages into the nerve. This is followed by destruction of the myelin. Fortunately, Schwann cells are not usually damaged; they are able to multiply and align themselves along the axon to form a new myelin sheath. This is an efficient and effective process, and full recovery can occur. In all but the mildest cases of GBS, there will be some damage to the underlying axon. This requires a longer recovery period, and when the axonal damage is more severe, recovery is often incomplete.

Axonal GBS requires a longer period of recovery and is more likely to result in some residual weakness.

Not all parts of the peripheral nervous system are affected equally in GBS. The nerve roots where they first emerge from the spinal cord and begin to become peripheral nerves seem to be the most susceptible, particularly the nerve roots containing the motor axons going to the muscles. Inflammation and degeneration of the myelin causes leakage of proteins from the blood into the CSF, causing the increased CSF protein concentration that characterizes the disease. The inflammation is usually restricted to the nerves and does not spill over into the CSF, although it is not altogether surprising that a few of these inflammatory cells do get into the CSF. The motor axons where they enter the muscle are also susceptible to early damage in GBS. It is this early and prominent involvement of the motor nerves that explains why weakness is a much more prominent symptom than loss of feeling in people with GBS.

CHAPTER 5

Supportive Treatments in the Acute Care Hospital

Treatment of GBS consists of supportive care and treatment of the underlying cause. This chapter discusses management of the effects of the disease rather than specific treatment of the cause. The progression of GBS can be divided into four phases. This chapter discusses the first two phases.

- The initial symptom, usually progressive weakness, and the process that leads to medical consultation and treatment, usually in a hospital.
- Early (acute) hospital care to initiate disease-specific treatment and prevent or treat complications of GBS.
- Rehabilitation that usually begins during the acute hospital stay, and often continues in a rehabilitation hospital or comparable setting.
- Long-term care, for the person with incomplete recovery.

WHY NEW GUILLAIN-BARRÉ SYNDROME PATIENTS ARE ADMITTED TO A HOSPITAL

The Patient at Risk

At the outset, it is difficult to predict with accuracy how severe a particular episode of GBS is going to be. During the first few days after the symptoms appear, it is impossible to confidently predict whether the GBS patient is going to remain only mildly inconvenienced, or is going to develop life-threatening weakness. Nor is it possible to predict whether the GBS patient will develop serious irregularities of heart rhythm or dramatic fluctuations in blood pressure. Therefore, immediate admission to a hospital and close monitoring of bodily functions is imperative for all people in whom the diagnosis of GBS is suspected, even if it has not yet been diagnosed. Anyone with GBS should be admitted to a facility that allows for constant monitoring of vital signs Close monitoring enables medical staff to recognize and respond quickly when deterioration becomes life threatening.

The early course of GBS is unpredictable. Breathing and circulation problems frequently develop, and close observation of the person with GBS is imperative.

Medical Staff

Supportive care for the person with GBS involves management of breathing, heart rhythm, blood pressure, and swallowing, as well as other important but not critical body functions, such as bowel and bladder control. Supportive care is also concerned with prevention and management of complications, such as infections, especially *pneumonia,* and blood clots. Several doctors will typically be involved in early care in all but the mildest cases. Depending on the needs of an individual patient, these may include a general or family doctor or internist, a neurologist, a pulmonary physician (a lung specialist, or *pulmonologist)* and a specialist in physical medicine and rehabilitation *(physiatrist).* Nursing care is very important in all cases of GBS. Ongoing treatment by physical and occupational therapists is usually needed.

Type of Hospital

The question as to what type of hospital to use may arise when considering acute care. Will the local community hospital suffice, or would a medical center/university hospital be preferable? Generally, most hospitals, including community hospitals, have an intensive care unit and the necessary physician specialists, particularly neurologists, pulmonologists, and physiatrists, who have treated GBS. They will know if the ICU and other community hospital facilities are capable of treating a GBS patient. An occasional patient may require prolonged ventilation, and daily meticulous care is important for a good outcome.

Therefore, it is not just the doctor's experience that can have an impact on the GBS patient, but also the quality and experience of the other professional staff, including nurses and physical, occupational, and respiratory therapists. The patient, family, and doctors may want to determine the appropriateness of the available hospital. Remember that a distant hospital will make visiting more difficult, and the patient's emotional wellbeing is an important part of his or her care. On the other hand, older patients with severe disease might benefit from care by a more experienced team, such as those found at specialized, state-of-the-art hospitals.

RESPIRATORY FAILURE

About 40 percent of GBS patients will develop some compromise in their breathing ability, and approximately 25 percent require artificial ventilation for some period of time. Frequent assessment of the patient's breathing, usually in an ICU, will help determine if breathing is failing sufficiently to warrant mechanical support. In some patients, breathing failure is so evident that simple bedside analysis indicates a need for ventilation. In others, development of breathing insufficiency may progress more slowly, and the decision to ventilate will be guided by various bedside breathing tests, as detailed below.

How Breathing Works

The *diaphragm* and intercostal muscles work together to expand the lungs and pull in air. The diaphragm is the major muscle of respiration. It is located just under the lungs, and is attached all around the lower part of the rib cage. It is shaped like a dome that bulges upward. It contracts or shortens during breathing in *(inspiration)* and descends to expand or enlarge the chest cavity and lungs. Breathing is also accomplished by the intercostal muscles, which are located between and attached to the ribs. Inspiration occurs when the intercostal muscles shorten or contract, and bring the ribs up and forward, to expand the chest and lungs. The air comes in through the nose or mouth and goes down the airway or trachea into the lungs. Oxygen passes from the air in the lungs into the blood that circulates through the lungs. If the nerves to the intercostal or diaphragmatic muscles are sufficiently damaged, the muscles will become weak, and the patient cannot take a deep enough breathe to maintain safe oxygen levels in the blood. Doctors can determine the amount of oxygen in the blood by measuring its pressure, which is normally over 60 millimeters of mercury (mm Hg). In healthy nonsmokers, this measurement is usually about 95+ mm Hg. The amount of oxygen can also be measured as its saturation in blood. A normal value in nonsmokers would be over 95 percent saturation. The oxygen level drops as breathing begins to get weaker.

The blood normally contains *carbon dioxide* (CO_2). The normal level of CO_2 in the bloodstream is approximately 35 to 40 mm Hg. During normal breathing the lungs exhale to eliminate CO_2 and prevent it from accumulating in the body. If breathing becomes weak, the next measurable evidence of poor breathing (after oxygen levels start to fall) is the accumulation of CO_2. Retained CO_2 causes the blood and other body fluids to become more acidic *(acidosis).* In this case, the CO_2 acts as a poison. Body chemistry depends on catalysts (protein chemicals, or *enzymes)* to enable metabolism. Enzymes maintain normal bodily functions, such as conversion of the food we eat into energy. These catalyst enzymes can no longer work effectively when the body becomes acidic. Metabolism, including brain function, deteriorates. The patient will not be able to think clearly and will become lethargic, a condition known as *CO_2 narcosis.* Eventually, the patient will stop breathing and suffocate. Obviously, retention of CO_2 is dangerous; it signals extremely poor breathing and is a clear sign that intervention is necessary. The goal of close monitoring of breathing function in GBS patients is to detect the earliest stages of breathing failure so that assisted ventilation can be started and the risks of oxygen deprivation and CO_2 narcosis can be avoided.

Close monitoring of breathing function in GBS patients is necessary to detect the earliest stages of breathing failure, so that assisted ventilation can be started and the risks of oxygen deprivation and CO_2 narcosis can be avoided.

Breathing Problems in GBS

Failure of breathing was the major cause of death in GBS patients prior to the 1950s, when the mortality rate was approximately 15 percent. The development in the late 1950s of modern mechanical ventilators to supply artificial respiration is primarily responsible for the decrease in mortality of GBS to its current rate of 3 to 5 percent. Patients are now more likely to die of the later complications of GBS, such as infections and blood clots. Failure of breathing is most often seen in conjunction with severe weakness of limb muscles, but occasionally it may occur with only mild weakness. Failure of breathing has also been described in patients with Miller Fisher syndrome. Thus, close monitoring is necessary, even if the patient does not seem to be severely weak.

GBS typically progresses over several days but occasionally develops extremely rapidly over hours. Therefore, it is imperative to closely monitor newly diagnosed GBS patients, even if their initial presentation reveals only mild weakness. Some people, especially smokers and former smokers, may have preexisting compromise of lung function. A person who has led a sedentary lifestyle may not even be aware of their impaired lung function. These patients need to be closely observed for deterioration of breathing.

Examination of Breathing

Assessment of breathing function usually begins at the time of admission to the hospital because breathing failure is a major risk in new GBS patients. The goal is first to determine the baseline breathing status, and then follow it closely so inadequate breathing can be identified early and treated. Several methods are available to monitor breathing. Patients should be asked if they feel breathless or have a sense of suffocation. Anxiety may cause similar symptoms, so objective signs of respiratory compromise should also be present before resorting to mechanical ventilation. Patients should be observed for signs of increased effort in breathing; patients who are struggling to breathe will usually perspire despite the coolness of the hospital environment. The number of times a person breathes each minute is called the *respiratory rate.* The respiratory rate is an extremely useful and simple measure of respiratory function that can be assessed at the bedside without complicated and expensive instruments. This rate is determined by watching or feeling the chest wall and counting the number of breaths. Usually the number of breaths in 15 seconds is counted, and the respiratory rate is then calculated by multiplying by four. The normal respiratory rate should be 10 to 15 per minute in a healthy adult. Patients who are having difficulty breathing will usually have a rapid pulse. This is easily measured. If the patient is in the ICU, the heart rate and respiratory rate can be continuously monitored electronically and shown on a display screen. The instruments can be set to predetermined levels so that if the breathing rate becomes too slow or too fast, an alarm is set off. Similarly, the alarm can be set to sound if the pulse becomes too fast or too slow. The patient's depth of inspiration is another useful marker of their breathing status; this can be assessed clinically, although it is less accurate than other methods. Breathing can be evaluated using the following methods:

- Count respiratory rate and estimate depth of breathing.
- Check oxygen level using pulse oximetry or arterial blood gas.
- Measure volume of a normal breath, tidal volume.
- Measure volume of a deep breath, vital capacity.
- Measure strength to inhale, inspiratory effort.
- easure speed to exhale, peak expiratory rate flow.

PULMONARY FUNCTION TESTS

Pulmonary function tests are used to test breathing. The preferred tests for the GBS patient are simple to administer and will minimize fatigue.

Tests for Breathing Effectiveness

A convenient indicator of the adequacy of breathing is the level of oxygen in the patient's blood; measured as the percentage of *oxygen saturation.* This percentage should be well into the upper 90s in healthy nonsmokers who have not had prior lung disease. Oxygen saturation can be easily monitored using a *pulse oximeter.* This device uses a lightweight plastic clip, or probe, that sits gently on the patient's fingertip. The probe is attached via a wire to a machine that continuously displays the percentage of saturation of the blood with oxygen on a display screen. The machine alarm is usually set so that low values will trigger a warning buzzer. Another test of blood oxygen level is the *arterial blood gas* (ABG). The ABG is the most accurate way of determining the level of oxygenation; it also measures the amount of CO2 in the blood. The ABG also measures the acid or alkaline nature of body chemistry, known as the *pH level.* The blood becomes more acidic as CO2 accumulates and O2 levels decline. Although the ABG is the most accurate measure of the efficiency of the lungs in taking in O2 and eliminating CO2, it does require the insertion of a needle into an artery, usually at the wrist or inner elbow, to remove a small amount of blood. The needle stick can be painful, usually more painful than drawing blood from a vein, as is done for most blood tests. The ABG is employed only when the additional information it provides is necessary to help guide patient management.

Breathing measurements may be repeated regularly, even hourly, in order to determine whether mechanical breathing support is necessary.

Testing of the Ability to Breathe

Several tests can measure the efficiency of the mechanics of breathing. These are essentially tests of the strength of the diaphragmatic and the intercostal muscles. These tests employ various instruments, which are easy to use at the bedside and with little difficulty for an exhausted patient. These *pulmonary function tests* are usually done at the time of the patient's admission to the hospital in order to determine the baseline status of their breathing. This baseline information may be particularly useful in people with preexisting or unrecognized lung disease, including smokers and other people who are inactive or have a sedentary lifestyle. They may have previously unrecognized pulmonary disease such as *chronic bronchitis* or *emphysema.* These initial tests will provide a baseline against which to compare further tests. Breathing measurements may be repeated regularly, even hourly, in order to determine whether mechanical breathing support is necessary.

There are four types of pulmonary function tests:

Tidal Volume

The *tidal volume* is the amount or volume of air moved by a patient with a single normal breath. It is measured in *liters* (1 liter equals approximately 1 quart).

Forced Vital Capacity

The vital capacity, often measured as the *forced vital capacity* (FVC), is the largest amount of air that a patient can force out of the lungs during strong exhalation after taking in a deep breath. To measure the FVC, the patient's lips are firmly wrapped around a tube or mouthpiece, and then they exhale as hard as possible. FVC is not always easy to measure. The test may give false readings if the patient tires or cannot firmly hold the mouthpiece with their lips. In small patients, such as children, and the obese, a FVC value based on body weight is used to help determine a role for mechanical ventilation.

Inspiratory Force

A person's ability to generate an *inspiratory force,* meaning to suck air into the lungs, is another method of evaluating breathing ability. This is another way of measuring the strength of the breathing muscles. This testing uses the same type of procedure as described for the FVC above except the patient is asked to breathe in as strongly as possible.

Breathing ability can be assessed by bedside examination supplemented by instrumental measurement of breathing and the amount of oxygen and carbon dioxide in the blood.

Expiratory Flow

The *expiratory flow rate* measures the speed at which air flows out of the lungs when a person forcibly exhales.

Most methods of testing air movement require the patient to grip the mouthpiece of the testing equipment firmly with their lips. If GBS has made the facial muscles weak, and the patient cannot maintain a good seal with their lips around the mouthpiece, then the test results may not be reliable. The tests are also tiring, and the GBS patient may have difficulty cooperating with the testing due to fatigue, even before overt weakness of the breathing muscles develops. The key is to combine clinical symptoms, observation of respiratory rate and depth, pulse rate, appearance of the patient (pallor and perspiration), oxygen saturation, and tests of mechanical efficiency of the breathing muscles in order to create an overall picture before making the decision to intervene with mechanical ventilation. It is better to err on the side of premature ventilation than to wait too long and have to initiate mechanical ventilation on an emergency basis.

Artificial/Mechanical Ventilation

Prompt initiation of mechanical ventilation is usually indicated if testing shows there is sufficient impairment of breathing. Once the decision to use mechanical ventilation is made, a flexible tube will be inserted into the patient's airway either through the mouth or the nose. This is called *intubation.* The procedure is performed as follows:

The patient is typically positioned flat on their back with their head tilted back. The throat is sprayed with local anesthetic to prevent gagging when the tube is passed down the throat. An instrument called a *laryngoscope* is inserted into the mouth and the back of the throat to inspect the back of the mouth and upper part of the throat (the *pharynx)* and the upper airway. An *endotracheal tube* is then passed through the nose or mouth and down into the windpipe *(trachea).* When the end of the tube reaches the trachea, a cuff at the inner end of the tube is inflated to secure it in place and create a gentle seal so air will only move in and out of the lungs and through the tube, not around it. An *Ambu bag* may be briefly attached to the outer end of the tube and squeezed by one person while a second person listens with a stethoscope over the lungs to assure that air is moving into both sides. The tube is then secured to the patient's face with tape and the outer end is connected to a mechanical ventilator. A chest x-ray is usually taken to assure proper placement of the tube in the airway.

Mechanical ventilation should be instituted when there is evidence of impending respiratory failure. It is tempting simply to add supplemental oxygen via the nose *(nasal cannula)* to address a patient's impaired breathing and lowered oxygen levels. However, this does not address weakening breathing muscles, and it supplies only temporary benefit. There is a natural aversion to putting a patient on mechanical ventilation, but delaying it can be life threatening. Continued weakening of breathing may warrant mechanical ventilation in spite of its invasiveness and potential risks. Furthermore, a sustained decrease in oxygenation can predispose the patient to irregular heartbeats *(arrhythmias* or *dysrhythmias),* which can be dangerous. Hence, there is added reason for frequent assessment of breathing function and early intervention with artificial ventilation if clinically indicated.

Risks of Mechanical Ventilation

Mechanical ventilation provides a ready solution to the problem of failure of breathing, but it should be remembered that it cannot fully replicate the natural way the body assures a clear airway and open lungs. For example, a ventilator cannot cough. Mechanical ventilation can predispose a patient to the development of a condition called *atelectasis,* which is the collapse of small segments of the lung, possibly leading to pneumonia. Mechanical ventilation carries additional risks. The endotracheal tube, when inserted, may be placed too far down the windpipe and into one of the two main bronchi, thus depriving the other lung of air. To address this issue, it is routine to obtain a chest x-ray after intubation in order to assure proper tube placement. Mechanical ventilation can also predispose a patient to lung collapse *(pneumothorax),* a condition in which air escapes from the lungs into the chest cavity. This complication is more likely in patients with preexisting lung disease, such as emphysema. Pneumothorax is usually treated with insertion of a tube through the chest wall into the lung cavity in order to expand the lung.

Mechanical ventilation is a relatively low-risk intervention that can be lifesaving for the GBS patient if their ability to breathe is deteriorating. Breathing difficulties can be managed without mechanical ventilation, but intubation is best planned as a deliberate, elective procedure rather than waiting until respiratory failure is imminent.

In order to help circumvent the inherent deficiencies of mechanical ventilation, various techniques are employed to help clear the lungs of secretions and prevent atelectasis and pneumonia. These methods remove excessive secretions by suction using a small plastic tube that is passed through the endotracheal tube into the lungs. Mini-nebulizer treatments can be used to administer aerosolized medications *(bronchodilators)* that will open the airways. These procedures are usually administered by a respiratory therapist or nurse who has been specially trained in care of the lungs.

Treatment of Mild Breathing Impairment

Patients with mildly compromised breathing may not necessarily require mechanical ventilation. However, they may be candidates for bronchodilators, mini-nebulizer therapy, and other treatments that can optimize lung function and reduce congestion. These include instructions on deep breathing and special *(segmental)* breathing exercises that ensure expansion of all parts of the lungs. Postural drainage may also be used. In this procedure, the patient is placed face down on the bed with their head hanging over the edge to facilitate optimal lung drainage. The respiratory therapist or nurse then manually claps on the patient's chest or vibrates the patient's chest in different areas to loosen accumulated mucus and help the patient clear these secretions by coughing. Sometimes a machine is used to provide this therapy.

The patient can be placed on mechanical ventilation if the clinical picture indicates a substantial risk of impending respiratory failure. Instituting mechanical ventilation as a planned procedure is much safer than doing it quickly during an emergency. Ultimately, the decision to initiate artificial ventilation is a clinical one. If a patient is showing obvious, rapid deterioration, the decision to intubate and ventilate may be easy to make. Perhaps more challenging to the treating physician is the patient who shows a slow deterioration or stable but borderline breathing capacity.

Prolonged Ventilator Use

The amount of time a GBS patient spends on a respirator may vary from as little as a few days to weeks, and in unusual cases, months. If the patient requires mechanical ventilation for more than 10 days to 2 weeks, the endotracheal tube will need to be replaced. The tube inserted through the nose or mouth can damage the pharynx, the voice box *(the larynx),* or the upper trachea if it is left in place for too long. This can lead to potential narrowing *(stenosis)* of the air passages and long-term breathing difficulties. If it becomes apparent that a patient is going to need mechanical ventilation for longer than approximately 2 weeks, a *tracheostomy* will be performed. This is a minor surgical procedure in which an incision is made at the base of the throat and a tube is inserted directly through the skin into the upper part of the trachea. The ventilator is then attached to the tracheostomy tube in the same way that it was attached to the endotracheal tube. It is possible to mechanically ventilate a patient through a tracheostomy for an indefinite period of time.

GBS patients who are weak enough to need long-term mechanical ventilation are prone to innumerable complications. They are more likely to get pneumonia. They are also prone to ulcerated tissue resulting from pressure *(bedsores)* and blood clots in the leg veins *(phlebitis).* It is also more difficult to maintain adequate nutrition and hydration.

If long-term mechanical ventilation is necessary, a tracheostomy will be performed in order to avoid damage to the structures of the upper airway. A strategy for enabling the patient to communicate will be essential because mechanical ventilation prevents verbal communication.

Communication Cards

The patient on a respirator cannot speak, and therefore will need alternate methods of communicating with hospital personnel and family. A pencil and paper on a clipboard can be used if the patient's hands are strong enough, but most GBS patients who require mechanical ventilation are too weak for this option. They can be instructed to use a simple code system, such as eye blinks or finger taps to signal "yes" or "no" responses. However, this method can become rapidly cumbersome and annoyingly slow; it is appropriate for short-term, simple communication, but it is unsatisfactory if mechanical ventilation is going to be needed for more than 2 weeks. As discussed in Chapter 2, a better alternative is a set of Communication Cards, which list common problems and issues that a GBS patient may want to discuss. These cards should be held up within the patient's field of vision so they can be seen easily.

Weaning

The mechanical support of ventilation will be continued until sufficient strength of the breathing muscles has returned. Almost all GBS patients eventually regain sufficient breathing capacity and can be removed from the ventilator. The process of gradually withdrawing the patient from mechanical ventilation is called *weaning.* Various signs and symptoms may provide a clue that the patient is ready to be weaned. For example, if the previously paralyzed patient begins to show head, neck, shoulder, and arm movement, the chest muscles of respiration may soon regain sufficient strength to consider a trial of weaning. The patient's ability to breathe provides a useful gauge of muscle strength, but it does not indicate the ability of the patient to sustain that effort. Accordingly, strength of inspiratory effort may not indicate the patient's ability to come off the respirator, but may signal the patient's ability to slowly start the weaning process. The purpose of gradual weaning is to demand more work of the breathing muscles so that strength and stamina can be slowly increased. The diaphragm loses its ability to function normally if it is not exercised regularly, and, as with any muscle, it becomes deconditioned when a person is on a mechanical ventilator. Gradual weaning forces the diaphragm to do increasingly demanding exercise until the patient is strong enough to breathe without assistance for hours at a time during the day. Removal of the airway tube *(extubation)* and detachment from the ventilator can then be planned. Two advantages of a tracheostomy are that breathing requires less effort and weaning is easier.

Weaning can be accomplished using the *intermittent mandatory ventilation* (IMV) setting on the mechanical ventilator. The IMV supplies a normal breath for a set number of times each minute, usually 10 to 12 times a minute. The patient may take additional breaths as they are able. As the strength and endurance of the patient's breathing muscles improve, the IMV rate can be lowered from 10 to 8, and lower. Thus, to continue to provide sufficient oxygen, the patient will need to take extra breaths. When the ventilator is set in "assist control mode," the machine delivers a full good breath every time a patient inhales, even if the patient's effort is weak. If the breathing rate falls below a selected back-up rate, the machine automatically delivers a sufficient breath at the selected rate.

A *T tube* is sometimes used later in the weaning process. This type of tube supplies a high oxygen flow rate, enabling the patient to get sufficient oxygen, even if the depth and rate of their breathing is low. The T tube is placed over the patient's tracheostomy tube for short periods of time, and is open to the atmosphere, so the patient is actually breathing unassisted. The T tube is used initially for only short periods of time according to the patient's clinical status. As the patient gets stronger, the duration of T tube use can be increased until eventually it can be used around the clock, indicating the patient's readiness for extubation.

Weaning is usually started during the day when the patient is awake and stronger. Normal individuals breathe less deeply when they are asleep, and therefore, when the patient is asleep, would be a poor time to attempt to wean a patient from ventilatory support. Most GBS patients show steady improvement after they plateau, and weaning tends to proceed steadily. Episodes of recurrent weakness are uncommon. However, fatigue may slow the weaning process, and patients with preexisting lung problems may take longer to be weaned. The longer a patient has been supported by mechanical ventilation, the longer weaning will take. Conversely, if a patient has been on the ventilator for only a few days, the weaning process is usually rapid.

A GBS patient who has required mechanical ventilation for more than a few days will need to be slowly weaned from ventilator support.

THE INTENSIVE CARE UNIT

Most of the non-GBS patients in the ICU are only there for a short stay. They may have had a heart attack or stroke, be postoperative, or have pneumonia with respiratory failure. Most GBS patients reach their maximum weakness within 2 weeks, and only about 25 percent will need mechanical ventilation; therefore, their ICU stay may also be short. However, an occasional patient may have a protracted stay because of a continued need for ventilatory support. These patients can be a challenge to even the most conscientious nurses and other caregivers. A protracted stay in the ICU can be difficult, especially if the patient experiences pain, hallucinations, and difficulties with communication. The support of family and friends is especially helpful in this situation.

Standards of Care

Medical personnel should follow the highest standards of care:

1. Provide close attention to the details of daily care, anticipate potential complications, and plan treatment interventions.
2. The weakest of patients can still hear and understand. Therefore, to help orient the patient and improve their comfort level, all personnel should introduce themselves and explain to the patient what they do and why they are there. All procedures should be explained in advance.
3. Present a positive, pleasant attitude and leave personal problems outside. Staff should show a caring and empathetic approach.
4. Supply constant reassurance that everything that can be done is being done.
5. Remember, most GBS patients make a full or nearly full recovery. Cautious optimism and honesty about the future will promote a positive attitude.
6. Keep the patient and their loved ones informed about the patient's status so they do not become frustrated or feel that they are being kept in the dark.

The ICU provides an optimal setting for the monitoring of vital signs, including circulation and breathing status. A kind, caring staff can help make a patient's ICU experience more bearable.

7. The patient may get confused about the date and time. Keep a clock and a calendar with the date circled daily in the room.
8. The pain experienced by GBS patients in the ICU and thereafter can be severe. Analgesics and other methods to reduce pain should be used liberally and frequently, as needed. Pain in GBS is very real. Do not unfairly conclude that the patient is merely hysterical.
9. Bowel and bladder problems are common. Staff should make sure the patient has adequate bowel and urine emptying and hygiene.
10. The patient and family may benefit from a better understanding of the disorder. Staff should direct family members to the GBS/CIDP Foundation International for information (see Resources).

BULBAR PALSY

Weakness of the muscles necessary for speech and swallowing is caused by damage to the lower cranial nerves, which are known as the *bulbar nerves.* They are designated by the Roman numerals IX, X, XI, and XII. *Bulbar palsy* results from weakness of the muscles supplied by these nerves. In isolation, bulbar palsy is uncommon in GBS, but it does occur in more severely affected patients. The bulbar nerves supply branches to the neck and throat, and enable normal swallowing, awareness of secretions in the throat, coughing, gagging, speech, and airway protection. Safe eating requires the normal functioning of the nerves that sense items in the throat, ensuring that food will go down the esophagus into the stomach and not into the windpipe. If the nerves that control eating are damaged, choking and gagging may occur, and aspiration of food or secretions into the lungs is possible. Methods to protect the patient's airway and supply safe, adequate nutrition are indicated. Bulbar palsy also causes slurred speech, making communication difficult.

Bulbar palsy causes speech and swallowing problems. Food or secretions may be aspirated into the lungs, causing pneumonia. Even if breathing is adequate, evidence of poor secretion handling may indicate the need to protect the airway with intubation.

Aspirating food or liquids down the airway into the lungs can result in *aspiration pneumonia,* a dangerous complication of bulbar palsy. When poor secretion handling is identified, the airway may need prompt protection either by frequent suctioning or by inserting an endotracheal tube that protects the airway, even though the patient may not be weak enough to need mechanical ventilation.

INVOLVEMENT OF OTHER CRANIAL NERVES

In addition to the bulbar nerves that come off the lower part of the brain, cranial nerves III through VII extend from the middle portion of the lower brain. They facilitate facial expression and eye closure (VII), chewing (V), and eye movement (III, IV, and VI). Weakness of the facial muscles is common in GBS, occurring in approximately 50 percent of cases. The patient may not be able to fully close their eyes when their facial muscles are weak, and saliva may drool from the corner of their mouth. They may appear expressionless and may be thought to be depressed. If eye closure is incomplete, the eyes may dry out and the clear and the outer layer of the eye (the *cornea)* may become ulcerated. It is sometimes necessary to tape the eyes closed during sleep and to moisten the eyes with artificial tears or ointment during wakefulness. Difficulty with chewing is very rare in GBS. Occasionally, weakness of chewing muscles is manifested as difficulty in keeping the mouth closed, and the weight of the jaw will make the mouth fall open and become dry. Weakness of the eye muscles will cause double vision and drooping of the upper eyelids. This may occur as part of typical GBS, or it may be the predominant feature in patients with Miller Fisher syndrome. Hearing is controlled by the eighth (VIII) cranial nerve, which is almost never involved in GBS. However, it has been described in a few patients, making it important to consider whether a patient on a ventilator appears unable to understand verbal communications. Cranial nerve I, the *olfactory* nerve necessary for the sense of smell, and cranial nerve II, the *optic* nerve necessary for vision, are not peripheral nerves, but are simply extensions of the brain. They are not affected in GBS.

AUTONOMIC NERVOUS SYSTEM DIFFICULTIES

The internal organs of the body are regulated in part by the autonomic nervous system (ANS), which functions automatically. Some parts of this system are located in the brain, but most of the nerves are located outside of the brain and spinal cord. These peripheral nerves can be damaged in GBS, leading to major internal organ problems. The ANS regulates many activities, including heartbeat, blood pressure, bowel motility, urinary/bladder function, kidney, and body chemistry and metabolic activities. The ANS includes two components: the *sympathetic* and *parasympathetic.* The sympathetic component prepares an individual for vigorous activity. For example, it raises the blood pressure and increases the heart rate. The parasympathetic component controls activities of the body such as gut motility and bladder function. The patient is usually not aware of many autonomic nerve activities because they do not cause symptoms; for example, elevated blood pressure as a normal response to physical exertion or pain. Some ANS functions may be apparent, such as increased perspiration with exertion.

ANS involvement in GBS is sometimes underappreciated, even by neurologists, yet the literature includes accounts of autonomic derangements that have caused major problems. Indeed, Landry's historical account of 10 patients from the late nineteenth century includes one that probably succumbed from irregular heartbeat *(cardiac arrhythmia).* Disturbances of autonomic nerves in GBS are usually more prominent in patients with more severe disease, especially those requiring mechanical ventilation. The risk of irregular or slow heartbeat is one of the reasons for monitoring newly-diagnosed patients closely in an ICU. The range of autonomic disturbances can vary in frequency and type. Several studies have demonstrated abnormalities affecting the heartbeat, with excessively slow, irregular, or rapid heartbeats, elevated or low blood pressure, urinary retention, and even low blood sodium levels. Most of these abnormalities become clinically evident during the patient's hospital care.

The autonomic nervous system regulates internal organ function. It can be affected in GBS, and needs to be closely monitored so that treatment can be instituted if necessary.

Heartbeat Irregularities

The heart beats normally at a rate of 60 to 100 times each minute, and the beat occurs at regular intervals. In patients with GBS, the heart may beat too slowly, too rapidly, or it may beat irregularly. The most common abnormality of heartbeat in GBS is sustained resting *tachycardia,* or rapid heartbeat. This is not, in itself, dangerous, but it is an indication of autonomic nerve involvement that may precede a more dangerous abnormality of cardiac rate or rhythm. Rapid heart rates of a degree sufficient to compromise the output of blood from the heart are much less common, but they do occur occasionally. Rates that remain consistently above 130 to 140 beats/minute can be dangerous. Increased heart rate is not necessarily due to autonomic involvement, but may reflect other problems, such as infection, fever, inadequate fluids *(dehydration),* or blood clots in the lungs *(pulmonary embolism).* In fact, these are more common causes of tachycardia in the GBS patient, and a careful search for these conditions should be made before attributing tachycardia to autonomic involvement. Treatment of tachycardia in GBS is seldom necessary, and any medical treatment should be used with great caution as it may lead to an abruptly slow heart rate *(bradycardia),* which is much more dangerous. It may be necessary to insert a temporary pacemaker to prevent bradycardia and maintain adequate cardiac output before treating tachycardia medically in GBS. Although bradycardia is uncommon in GBS, it can develop. Rates that stay consistently below 40 to 50 beats/minute are potentially dangerous. An excessively slow heartbeat may necessitate medical treatment with drugs.

Cardiac arrhythmia can also occur in GBS. As with a tachycardia, it is important to consider other causes before attributing arrhythmia to an effect on the ANS. Reduced oxygenation of the blood due to respiratory failure, pulmonary emboli, electrolyte imbalance, and infection can all cause cardiac arrhythmia. If a GBS patient has an irregular cardiac rhythm, inadequate oxygenation due to problems with breathing may exacerbate the arrhythmia, potentially turning a benign arrhythmia into a life-threatening situation. Thus, meticulous management of ventilatory failure and early mechanical ventilation are doubly important in patients with cardiac arrhythmia.

The GBS patient is at risk of developing an irregular, slow, or rapid heartbeat. This is most often due to infection or respiratory failure, but it may result from a direct effect of GBS on the autonomic nervous system. Careful monitoring is needed in most instances, but treatment with medication or a pacemaker may be required.

Low Blood Pressure

Blood pressure (BP) measurement consists of two numbers. The upper number, the *systolic pressure,* is normally between 110 and 140, and is measured as a pressure in millimeters of mercury (mm Hg). The lower number, the *diastolic pressure,* is usually 60 to 90 mm Hg. When blood pressure is affected by autonomic nervous system abnormalities in GBS, it almost always affects the systolic pressure. Systolic blood pressure below 90 to 100 mm Hg is referred to as *hypotension.* Low blood pressure is relatively common in GBS, and can be dangerous. Frequently, it is only apparent when the patient changes posture from a lying position to a sitting or standing position, and it is therefore called *postural hypotension.* This commonly results from a lack of oxygen, a pulmonary embolism, infection, or dehydration, but it can also result from autonomic failure. Low blood pressure resulting from autonomic failure will resolve as the patient's overall health improves.

There are various treatments for low blood pressure. The patient should first be placed in a horizontal position to minimize the pooling of blood in the leg veins. If this is insufficient, it may be necessary to lower the head of the bed so that the legs are higher than the heart. However, this is an uncomfortable position that should be used only for short periods of time. Antiembolism (elastic) stockings, such as TEDs®, can be worn to reduce the pooling of blood in the legs; this is particularly important when the patient first gets up from bed after a period of confinement. Intravenous fluid hydration can be used to expand blood volume when the blood volume is reduced because of dehydration. It is also useful for short-term treatment of hypotension due to autonomic failure. Hypotension almost never needs treatment with medication, and drugs should be used with great caution. Blood pressure can rise rapidly when treated, and there is the risk that it will rise too high. In the majority of people with GBS, hypotension is no more than a mild nuisance—the patient simply feels a bit dizzy or lightheaded in the upright position. Oral medications can be used if the hypotension is severe and prolonged. Options include fludrocortisone acetate (Florinef®) a drug that causes salt and fluid retention, leading to increased intravascular volume and higher blood pressure. Midodrine (ProAmatine®) stimulates the sympathetic nerves to the blood vessels and increases their tone, leading to reduced pooling of blood and raising the blood pressure. In extremely rare instances of severe hypotension, dopamine can be given to support blood pressure. It is critical to aggressively seek an explanation other than autonomic nerve involvement if hypotension is so severe that medication is needed to maintain the blood pressure in a safe range.

High Blood Pressure

Some degree of elevated blood pressure *(hypertension)* may occur in as many as 50 percent of patients with GBS. The illness and the anxiety that accompanies it may also exacerbate preexisting hypertension. The degree of hypertension is usually mild and short lived, often interspersed with periods of low blood pressure. There are very few negative consequences of short periods of moderate hypertension to levels of 180 to 200 mm Hg systolic or even higher. If the patient is older and has preexisting cardiac disease or has had a stroke in the past, the risk of complications from hypertension is greater and treatment should be instituted sooner. Brief periods of hypertension should not be treated, but if the blood pressure is sustained above 200 mm Hg systolic for several hours, treatment should be considered. The risk of treatment is that catastrophic hypotension may suddenly develop, and it may be very difficult to reverse. If treatment is deemed necessary, simple maneuvers, such as elevation of the head of the bed, are often sufficient. Remove compression stockings if the patient is wearing them. If that is ineffective, small doses of a diuretic such as furosemide (Lasix®) can be helpful. If more potent medications are needed, short-acting forms should be used so that the effects can be rapidly reversed if the blood pressure falls too low.

Postural hypotension, sustained hypertension, and fluctuation between high and low blood pressure may occur in GBS. In rare instances, specific medical treatment may be needed, but most patients need only simple, nonpharmacological strategies or no treatment at all.

Urination

Difficulty passing urine is common in GBS, particularly in older men with prostate enlargement, who may have difficulty urinating while lying down. Less commonly, retention of urine may occur with partial or complete inability to empty the bladder. Bladder stimulants are seldom helpful; they can cause a lot of pain in the area of the bladder and should be avoided. It is probably better to pass a catheter into the bladder if difficulty with urination develops, so that the urine can be continuously drained into a bag. The risk of having a catheter in the bladder is that infection can develop, but this is not usually a problem in the short term; the risk is usually outweighed by the convenience.

Decreased Intestinal Activity

Impaired function of the ANS can cause slowed intestinal motility. The most common manifestation of impairment is constipation. Delayed emptying of the stomach into the small intestine and uncomfortable bloating can occur, but this is rare. Constipation can be particularly bothersome. Simple immobility can reduce bowel motility, leading to constipation. Reduced food, fluid, and fiber intake, or even a change from a familiar diet can result in constipation. Pain and other medications can contribute to reduced bowel motility. A variety of methods can be used to treat constipation, including simple measures such as milk of magnesia, stool softeners, such as docusate sodium (Colace®), or other agents, such as psyllium (Metamucil®). Some agents not originally designed for constipation, such as lactulose (Chronulac®), can be used. A suggested starting dose is 3 tablespoons (45 cc) four times a day until the patient has a bowel movement, then 1 to 3 tablespoons daily. A powdered version of lactulose (MiraLax®) can be mixed with a liquid of choice, such as juice, making it more palatable than lactulose, a rather sweet liquid. Senna is a natural vegetable derivative that is available in a tablet form, as granules, or as syrup. It usually generates a bowel movement within 6 to 12 hours. The gentle action and minimal side effects of senna make it a popular laxative.

Constipation is a common problem for the hospitalized patient, and GBS may further exacerbate this potential problem. Constipation can be treated by a variety of methods.

Low Blood Salt Level

The normal blood sodium level is 135 to 145 units. Approximately 20 percent of GBS patients develop a decreased level of sodium in their bloodstream. The decrease is usually very mild and does not need treatment. The cause may relate to excessive secretion of an antidiuretic hormone that conserves water in the body by decreasing urine output. It may also relate to abnormal functioning of the ANS. Some drugs may also lower the blood concentration of sodium. A rapid fall in sodium, or a very low sodium level (below 120), may result in confusion or even seizures. Several treatments are available to raise sodium levels. Restriction of fluid intake may be all that is needed. Other treatments options include the use of strong diuretics, medications to generate an increased urine output, such as furosemide (Lasix®), intravenous administration of salt (saline) solutions, urea, and the use of antibiotics, such as demeclocycline.

Low blood salt levels are an uncommon complication of GBS and may be related to autonomic failure. This condition can be treated.

BLOOD CLOTS

The Development and Consequences of Blood Clots

Blood flow in the veins of the legs and the pelvis tends to be slow in patients confined to bed, especially if they are paralyzed or weak. Inactivity and the resulting stagnation of venous blood flow can lead to development of leg swelling *(edema)* and the formation of blood clots *(thrombi)* in the deep veins. This condition is called *deep venous thrombosis.* These clots can become enlarged, break off, and travel to the lungs, where they are called *pulmonary emboli.* A large clot in the lungs can block the flow of blood, and the lungs will not be able to provide oxygen for the body. Blood clots in the lung can also block blood from flowing to the heart. Poor oxygenation and decreased blood flow to the heart can lead to shock and death. Obviously it is important to try to prevent such potential catastrophes.

Preventing Blood Clots

Several methods are available to reduce the risk of blood clot formation. Common methods include the use of *anticoagulants* (blood thinners), intermittent limb compression, antiembolism stockings, frequent changes of position, and limb movement or mobilization. Table 5-1 lists various methods to reduce the risk of developing blood clots.

The recommended anticoagulant is heparin, which is available in two forms. Both forms are administered as injections under the skin *(subcutaneous* injections). *Unfractionated heparin* is an older form of heparin. The newer heparins are called *low molecular weight heparins* (LMWHs). The LMWHs may be more effective, but they are more expensive than the older, unfractionated heparin.

In limb compression, inflatable cuffs are wrapped around the calves and thighs. These cuffs are intermittently inflated to squeeze the legs, providing a pumping action that facilitates the movement of the blood through the veins of the legs. Obviously, this cannot be used for the pelvic veins, where many clots are formed. Intermittent limb compression probably also reduces clot formation by altering blood chemistry.

Anti-embolism stockings may reduce clots by obliterating the superficial veins of the legs, thereby increasing the blood flow through the deeper veins where the clots form. In other words, the faster the flow, the less likely clots will form. Early movement *(ambulation),* as in walking, can also reduce the risk of clot formation, but in GBS, this approach is usually limited by paralysis. Regular changes of position and passive movement of the limbs can also limit clot formation. Leg swelling usually indicates excessive water is accumulating in the calf. This can also be a sign of blockage of the veins with clots, but it can also be related to immobility. Edema can be relieved by leg elevation with the feet positioned above the knees, anti-embolism stockings, or intermittent limb compression.

Table 5-1 Methods to Reduce Risk of Blood Clot Formation

- Anti-embolism (elastic) stockings
- intermittent leg compression (intermittent pneumatic limb compression)
- Frequent repositioning of a paralyzed patient
- Passive movement of paralyzed limbs
- Early mobilization
- Anticoagulants (subcutaneous heparin injections)

The paralyzed patient is at increased risk of developing blood clots in the deep veins of the legs. These clots may break free and travel to the lungs, causing pulmonary embolism, a dangerous condition. Lowdose subcutaneous heparin should be administered, and physical means of increasing deep venous blood flow should be employed.

Identification and Treatment of Blood Clots

Clinical findings that raise suspicion of the development of deep venous thrombosis include swelling and pain in a calf or thigh. If they are large enough, clots can usually be identified by an *ultrasound imaging study* combined with *Doppler flow analysis* of the blood flowing in the veins. Using the combination of these two modalities is called a *duplex study.*

Patients who develop blood clots should be treated with anticoagulants. As discussed above, low-dose heparin in administered subcutaneously to prevent clots from forming. If blood clots develop despite this prophylactic treatment, more aggressive anticoagulant treatment is necessary. This initially consists of intravenous infusion of much higher doses of heparin, followed by longer term treatment with the oral anticoagulant warfarin (Coumadin®). Heparin acts quickly, providing protection against further clot formation within hours. Warfarin typically takes days to provide protection against further clot formation, so heparin needs to be continued until blood tests show that the warfarin is fully effective. As long as a patient continues to take warfarin, regular blood tests are needed to ensure that the degree of anticoagulation is appropriate. The time it takes for the patient's blood to clot in a test tube is measured and compared with a standard time in order to derive an *international normalized ratio* (INR) to determine proper dosing. The INR is usually maintained at a value of 2 to 3. For the occasional patient in whom anticoagulants are contraindicated, such as a patient with an actively bleeding stomach ulcer or some other bleeding problem, an alternative method to protect the lungs from clots is the use of a filter. Using a tube or catheter, this metal device is inserted through the femoral vein in the groin and is passed into the main vein that drains the legs, the *inferior vena cava* (IVC). This filter resembles an umbrella without a cloth cover. It blocks large clots arising from the leg veins into the IVC. These clots will be trapped by the filter until the natural metabolism of the body can dissolve them.

Once blood clots have formed, more aggressive anticoagulation is needed, beginning with high-dose intravenous heparin followed by oral warfarin. If anticoagulants cannot be used, an IVC filter can be placed to prevent the blood clots from reaching the lungs.

NUTRITION AND HYDRATION

GBS patients may have difficulty maintaining adequate nourishment and hydration. Patients using mechanical ventilation will be unable to swallow normally because of interference from the endotracheal tube. Patients with bulbar palsy also have a limited ability to swallow because the muscles that coordinate the complex act of swallowing are weak. Failed attempts to swallow may result in food and fluids being aspirated into the lungs. To complicate matters further, hospitals, particularly the ICU, are dry, warm places, causing fluid loss through evaporation from both the skin and lungs and through sweating. Infections resulting in increased body temperature can increase the loss of fluid. Infections also increase the metabolic demands of the body. Seriously ill and often depressed patients may resist attempts to maintain adequate food and fluids. All of these factors conspire to create malnutrition and dehydration if great care is not taken.

If the patient cannot safely take food and fluids by mouth, or is completely unable to do so, alternative strategies for feeding will need to be considered. Fluid balance can be maintained by intravenous administration for the first few days. However, if the patient continues to be unable to take in food and liquid, other strategies will have to be devised. The dehydrated and malnourished patient is at increased risk or infection, edema, and skin breakdown, leading to bedsores—especially in places where the bones lie directly under the skin.

Feeding Options

The symptoms of drooling, gagging, and choking in bulbar palsy indicate that eating should be stopped and further assessment performed. An evaluation can be conducted by a speech pathologist, perhaps including an x-ray study that assesses swallowing *(video swallow study).* Sometimes a simple bedside evaluation will indicate the need for a feeding tube. If a swallowing study shows evidence of aspiration or unreliable swallowing, or if the patient is intubated, feeding can be accomplished using a *nasogastric* feeding tube. This tube is passed through the nose and down the throat into the stomach. Liquid nutrition is supplied through the tube. The caloric need will increase if the patient is feverish. A nasogastric tube can be left in place for a few weeks, but if long-term nutrition needs are anticipated, a tube will need to be inserted directly into the stomach through the abdominal wall. This procedure involves passing a tube through the mouth and down into the stomach. Then the stomach is inflated with a small amount of air. Under local anesthetic, a small incision is made in the abdominal wall and a second tube is inserted into the inflated stomach and secured in place. The first tube is then removed. This procedure is known as a *percutaneous gastrostomy* the tube used is called a) *PEG tube.* The PEG tube can be used indefinitely for fluid and nourishment needs, and can be removed when the patient is able to take food by mouth safely.

An inability to maintain sufficient food and fluid intake is common in severe GBS. The earliest fluid requirements can be given intravenously, but nourishment needs to be started within a week through a stomach tube. A PEG tube will be needed if long-term tube feeding is anticipated.

Nutrition Alternatives/Caloric Needs

GBS patients may require 1,500 to 2,000 or more calories each day. Several commercial products are available for tube feeding, including Ensure Plus®, Jevity®, Resource®, and Glucerna® for diabetics and Pulmocare® for respirator patients. A high-fiber product is recommended in order to minimize problems with constipation in patients who are tube fed. Feedings are usually started at a low rate of administration in combination with water. Patients with an infection, such as pneumonia, may have higher caloric requirements, up to 3,000 calories each day. It is usually difficult to weigh a paralyzed patient in bed, especially one on a ventilator, so monitoring weight can be difficult. It is preferable in the short term to provide an excess of calories from both protein and nonprotein sources in order to avoid weight loss of more than 10 percent of body weight and loss of muscle mass. Guidance by a dietician or nutritionist is critical in determining caloric needs. The patient may develop diarrhea when tube feeding is started, so the product should be diluted at first.

Hydration

The fluid needs of normal people are dealt with automatically by thirst. However, the paralyzed patient does not have the ability to respond to the thirst stimulus. Accordingly, caregivers must make sure the patient takes in adequate water. Humans, like most biologic systems, are approximately 70 percent water, so adequate hydration is of utmost importance. In the hospital setting, nurses typically tally a patient's fluid intake by mouth and the intravenous route, and also the output through the urine. People typically lose an additional 700 cc (3/4 of a quart) of water per day through evaporation from their skin. This is known as *insensible loss,* and even though this is not measurable, it also has to be replaced. Insensible fluid loss is increased by fever, rapid breathing, and by merely being in the warm, dry climate of an ICU. Early in the course of severe GBS, patients who cannot safely swallow can be given water as an intravenous fluid; for example, 5 percent dextrose in water (D5W), 5 percent dextrose in half-normal saline solution (0.45 percent salt in water) (D5 1/2 normal saline), or 5 percent dextrose (a form of sugar) in normal saline solution (0.9 percent salt solution) (D5 normal saline). Dextrose is a sugar that supplies some calories, and it is mixed in a solution of water or salt. Supplements, including potassium and multivitamins, may be added as clinically indicated. If the blood salt level falls, the concentration of sodium in the intravenous fluid can be increased. Depending upon the patient's clinical status, 90 to 110 cc of fluid solution each hour may be needed by intravenous administration. The amount of intravenous fluid replacement can be proportionately decreased if the patient is fed via a nasogastric or PEG tube.

Adequate hydration and nutrition are important for the GBS patient, who may have a higher caloric requirement than normally expected. If the patient has a fever, water loss and perspiration will further increase fluid requirements.

The hydration status of the patient can be assessed by measuring the daily intake and output of fluids (the *I/O chart),* examining the moisture of the skin, measuring blood chemical composition, and measuring the blood concentration of hemoglobin. The color of the urine can be examined, and the *specific gravity* (a measure of urine concentration) can be measured.

PREVENTION OF INFECTION

Risks for Pneumonia

The immobilized patient is particularly vulnerable to infections for several reasons, and it is prudent to take steps to try to reduce this potential complication of GBS. Pneumonia can occur from poor air movement in and out of the lungs. As noted above, mechanical ventilation is artificial and cannot fully duplicate normal breathing. It blunts the mechanisms that normal people use to prevent lung infection, such as coughing to clear secretions. If the lower cranial nerves are damaged (as in bulbar palsy), the throat sensations and reflex muscle activity that protect the airway will be compromised. The protective reflex closure of the upper airway at the throat may be decreased, allowing liquids to enter the trachea and lungs. Infection of the upper respiratory tract is the most common trigger of GBS, and patients may suffer residual effects of the antecedent infection when the paralytic phase develops, further increasing the risk of pneumonia. GBS patients with clinically inactive lung disease, especially smokers with chronic bronchitis or emphysema, are also at increased risk to develop pneumonia.

Prevention of Pneumonia

Several methods are available to help keep the lungs open, clear secretions, and reduce the risk of pneumonia. Collapse of small segments of the lung tissue (atelectasis) can readily occur if breathing is shallow. This is often the precursor of pneumonia. Methods to reduce this complication include various respiratory therapy techniques. A fine mist of medications that dilate or enlarge the upper airway can be administered. Using this mini-nebulizer method of administering bronchodilators, liquid medication is placed in a plastic bottle and attached to a mist producer. The patient holds the mouthpiece of the device with their lips and the medication is delivered as a mist into the lungs as they inhale. In addition, should the patient develop excessive secretions, the nurse or respiratory therapist can pass a flexible narrow tube down the throat to remove these unwanted and dangerous liquids by suction. Chest physical therapy, which involves clapping on various parts of the chest wall, can help to loosen secretions and mobilize them, making it easier to remove them by coughing. As discussed previously, the patient can be placed face down with their head hanging over the edge of the bed so that gravity can help drain secretions. Prophylactic treatment with antibiotics to prevent infection is very rarely indicated because this can foster the development of resistant strains of bacterial infections.

Pneumonia and Antibiotics

The GBS patient in the ICU, whether being supported by mechanical ventilation or not, needs to be closely monitored for pneumonia. A chest x-ray is usually done at the time of admission to the hospital in order to evaluate the baseline status of the lungs; this may also reveal unsuspected chronic bronchitis. The chest will be carefully examined every day with a stethoscope, and the temperature will be closely monitored, usually several times each day, to look for early signs of infection. The chest x-ray will be repeated if there are clinical features that suggest the development of pneumonia. Secretions from the lungs obtained by coughing or by suction will be examined for signs of infection, and be cultured in the laboratory to see if any microorganisms are present. If there is an abnormal growth of bacteria, the laboratory will test its sensitivity to different antibiotics. The signs of pneumonia include fever, increased respiratory distress, increased production of secretions (including a change in consistency and color), and increased crackling sounds that can be heard over the chest with a stethoscope. Antibiotics will be started immediately if pneumonia is diagnosed. A pulmonologist or infectious disease consultant will often be consulted because such a specialist is more familiar with the organisms that produce common hospital-acquired pneumonias. The antibiotic may be changed, however, once the result of the sputum culture and sensitivity are available. In some instances, a fever may develop with no identifiable source of infection. In such cases, the doctors may assume that it is a pulmonary infection, but they will have to treat the infection without full knowledge of the infecting organism, and therefore which antibiotic is best. Choice of antibiotic in such situations will be based on the most likely cause of the infection. Physical therapy for the chest, nebulizer treatments, bronchodilator medications, and medications that help to liquefy secretions *(expectorants)* can also help clear chest infections.

Bladder Infections and Hygiene

Urinary tract infection is another risk for the GBS patient. Urine may stagnate in the bladder and become infected if the patient has weakness of the bladder muscles due to autonomic involvement. This risk may be increased if a catheter is in place. Risk of urinary tract infection is decreased if a high flow of urine is maintained, so administration of sufficient fluids to maintain high urine output is important. GBS patients must be closely monitored for signs of urinary tract infection. It is important to remember that the typical symptoms of urinary tract infection, including increased frequency of urination and a burning feeling when urine is passed, may be absent in GBS patients and, of course, will not be present if the patient is catheterized. The urine should be examined for cloudiness and odor because increased sediment and a strong odor are indicators of possible infection. The urine should also be checked regularly using a small strip of paper impregnated with various chemicals that can detect blood or increased protein, which are further indications of possible infection. If the patient is not catheterized, the urine will seldom be sent to the laboratory to be checked for infection unless there are indicators of infection. If there is a catheter in place, a specimen will be sent from time to time to ensure that there is no abnormal bacterial growth. Urinary tract infection is another possible cause of fever, and the feverish patient should routinely have their urine checked for signs of infection.

Occasionally, especially in the severely weak GBS patient who has an intravenous line, an endotracheal tube or tracheostomy, and a bladder catheter, infection can spread to the blood, a condition called *septicemia.* Infection may spread to other organs if septicemia develops. This is an extremely serious, often life-threatening condition that requires urgent treatment, usually with multiple antibiotics. Indications that an infection has developed into septicemia include high fever, rapid heart rate, and low blood pressure. The patient may become confused, and urine output may drop. In such situations, a blood sample will be taken to see if there are bacteria circulating in the blood. The sample will be sent to a laboratory, where attempts will be made to identify the infectious organism. This is a medical emergency, and treatment should not await the identity of the specific organism. Antibiotics can be changed once the organism has been identified.

Infection is a common complication of GBS, usually involving the lungs and the bladder. Patients should be closely monitored for signs of infection, and antibiotics administered when appropriate.

BRAIN AND SPINAL CORD COMPLICATIONS, CONFUSION, AND HALLUCINATIONS

Complications of GBS involving the brain and spinal cord can result in abnormal functioning of the brain, sometimes leading to diagnostic uncertainty. These complications include the following.

Optic Neuritis and Papilledema

The optic nerve is the nerve that enables us to see. Light entering the eye activates nerve cells in the retina, and these cells send the visual information to the brain through the optic nerve. The optic nerve is not a true peripheral nerve, but rather an extension of the central nervous system. It should not be affected by GBS, but on very rare occasions, the same inflammation and demyelination that affects the peripheral nerves may also damage the optic nerve, a condition called *optic neuritis.* On the extremely rare occasions when this does happen, it affects only one eye. There will be blurred vision or even complete loss of vision in the affected eye, and pain will be felt behind the eye. A magnetic resonance image (MRI) of the brain may be ordered if optic neuritis is suspected. Treatment of optic neuritis usually entails the administration of highdose, intravenous steroids for 3 to 5 days. The prognosis is good and full return of vision is to be expected. The optic nerve may also swell, a condition known as *papilledema.* Although more common than optic neuritis, papilledema is also rare, occurring in perhaps 5 percent of patients. It is a little more common in children. Papilledema usually affects both eyes and causes mild blurring of vision. Papilledema can be recognized by looking into the back of the eye with an ophthalmoscope. Although this condition is not due to direct damage to the optic nerve, its exact cause is unknown. Papilledema usually occurs in patients with high spinal fluid protein levels. It has been suggested that impaired absorption of spinal fluid may contribute to swelling. However, papilledema occasionally occurs in patients with only mildly elevated cerebrospinal fluid (CSF) protein levels, so this explanation is questionable. Papilledema improves and resolves completely with time and without specific treatment.

Temporary impairment of vision is an uncommon but known complication of GBS, possibly resulting from papilledema or optic neuritis.

Mental Confusion

Impairment of higher brain functions—as indicated by drowsiness, confusion, disorientation, and sluggish, inaccurate thinking and speech—may occur in GBS and is called encephalopathy. Seizures may occur, but this is extremely rare. These changes are not due to injury of nerves in the brain from immune system attack. The most common cause is impaired blood oxygen supply resulting from weakness of the muscles of respiration. Immediate attention should be given to the respiratory status of a patient who becomes confused. Diligent monitoring of breathing function and oxygenation can usually prevent this difficulty. Retention of carbon dioxide from impaired breathing can cause *encephalopathy,* which can also be prevented with diligent attention to proper breathing support.

Sedatives and narcotic pain medications can also contribute to confusion. Low blood sodium level, mediated by excessive body retention of water via the kidneys, can also cause confusion, especially if the sodium level drops below 120 units (mEq/liter). Infection also needs to be considered. Elderly patients with GBS are particularly prone to developing encephalopathy. Inflammatory demyelination of peripheral nerves and the central nervous system has been reported in children and adults, but this is rare. Central nervous system (CNS) inflammation and demyelination may affect the brain, resulting in encephalitis, or the spinal cord (transverse myelitis), and when both are affected, the condition is called *encephalomyelitis.*

ICU Psychosis and Hallucinations

Confusion in the GBS patient in the ICU may also be due to psychosis. Multiple factors can contribute to this, including isolation, anxiety, and loss of awareness of day and night with disturbance of the sleep cycle. Patients become confused and agitated, and often experience vivid hallucinations. The hallucinations may be relatively benign and more curious than scary, such as seeing mice running up and down the blinds. They can also be morbid and frightening. Some hallucinations have a basis in reality because the frequent abnormal sensations experienced by GBS patients are misinterpreted by the brain.

It is important to determine whether a patient's confusion represents an emotional reaction to prolonged confinement or is the result of encephalopathy, so that appropriate treatment can be provided. If the GBS patients may develop signs of central confusion is the result of encephalopathy, treatment of the underlying cause (lack of oxygen, low blood sodium, or a reaction to medication) is indicated. If the confusion is the result of psychosis, constant reassurance, family contact, and access to familiar objects may be sufficient. However, medication may be needed for short periods. Prognosis for ICU psychosis is excellent, and patients do not have an increased risk for subsequent psychiatric problems.

GBS patients may develop signs of central nervous system involvement, most often caused by lack of oxygen, inflammatory demyelination in the brain, or psychosis. Confusion and hallucinations are common in GBS and should be treated.

EARLY REHABILITATION AND PREVENTION OF THE COMPLICATIONS OF IMMOBILIZATION

Rehabilitation of the GBS patient begins at the earliest practical time after admission to the hospital. Innumerable aspects of care fall under the umbrella of rehabilitation. Indeed, until the advent of treatments directed at stabilizing the presumed abnormalities of the immune system that underlie GBS, rehabilitation was the only treatment available. Physical and occupational therapy remain essential components of GBS care. A rehabilitation program is typically orchestrated under the guidance of a physiatrist. Some methods of rehabilitation and supportive care for the new GBS patient are listed in Table 5-2. Several specialists may participate in rehabilitation, including a physical therapist, occupational therapist, and others. The weaker the patient, the more likely rehabilitative care will contribute to a reduction in the complications of paralysis and lead to improvement. The rehabilitation process will continue in a rehabilitation hospital after discharge, depending on the severity of the patient's weakness and the pace of recovery.

Table 5-2. Highlights of Rehabilitation in the Acute Care Hospital

- Range of motion exercises to reduce risk of muscle shortening (contractures)
- Positioning limbs to reduce risk of nerve compressions
- Splints to reduce tendon shortening

Rehabilitation interventions in the acute care setting typically involve methods to address problems unique to the paralyzed or severely weakened patient. After discharge to a rehabilitation center, further therapy care will be provided to help the patient return to independent and, hopefully, normal functioning.

Nerve Compression

The paralyzed patient is prone to excessive pressure at certain areas of the body, which can compress and injure underlying nerves. This problem is accentuated in prolonged paralysis by loss of muscle mass and the subcutaneous fat that usually provides padding to protect the nerves. The two nerves that are at the greatest risk for injury of this type are the *peroneal* and *ulnar* nerves. The peroneal nerve lies just under the skin where it crosses the outer aspect of the knee, crossing over the fibular bone. The ulnar nerve crosses the inside of the elbow just under the skin. At both of these sites, the nerve is prone to compression between the mattress and the underlying bone. Peroneal nerve injury is particularly common in the paralyzed patient. The weight of the leg, caused by lying on the back, presses the nerve against the bone, resulting in additional damage to that already caused by GBS. Damage to the peroneal nerve causes footdrop, and some of the residual footdrop in GBS patients may be partly related to this added compressive peroneal neuropathy. Less commonly, the ulnar nerve is damaged by pressure of the inside of the arm against the mattress. This causes numbness along the inside of the hand and weakness of some of the hand muscles. These nerves may also be compressed by cuffs placed around the limb, as is commonly done to prevent blood clots. Care must be taken to ensure that the cuff is placed in such a way that it does not compress the nerve. Meticulous nursing care is the best way to prevent nerve compression injuries. An air mattress essentially eliminates this type of complication. However, if the patient is in a regular bed, frequent turning and repositioning is essential. Soft lamb's wool elbow pads can be used to protect the ulnar nerves.

Bedsores (Pressure Sores or Decubiti)

Some areas of the body have relatively small amounts of soft tissue between the skin and underlying bone, especially at bony prominences. Due to the limited amount of soft tissue between the skin and bone, these areas do not absorb pressure well, and the overlying skin has a greater risk of breaking down and becoming ulcerated. The risk of skin breakdown is greater if the patient is paralyzed or in bed for prolonged periods. Once a bedsore develops, it can be extremely difficult to heal, so prevention is critical. Areas at particular risk for bedsores include the heels, lower back *(sacral)* area, buttocks, over the hips, outer ankles, and ears.

Prevention of Bedsores

A paralyzed patient should be cared for on an air mattress whenever possible. This will essentially eliminate the risk of bedsores. Egg crate foam mattresses and sheepskins also reduce the risk of skin breakdown. If a patient with reduced movement, even if not fully paralyzed, is on a regular mattress, frequent repositioning and padding of areas prone to pressure injuries are the basis of the prevention. A thick foam or sheepskin pad under the heels and around the feet can be used. Alternatively, the weight of the leg can be intermittently supported by a pillow or foam pad under the calf to keep the heel completely off the mattress. Heel pads should be right angle–shaped and held in place with a Velcro® strap. Another method is the Multi-Podus® splint, described below in the section on treatment of foot-drop. This type of splint simultaneously takes the weight off the heel and cradles the foot and leg. It is important that nurses take the time and make the effort to communicate with the patient about pain and pressure, and explain the need for protective padding. Some patients will experience discomfort at areas of excessive pressure. However, GBS patients may have reduced sensation and may not develop discomfort at pressure sites, making regular inspection of high-risk areas essential.

Inspecting High-Risk Areas for Skin Breakdown

The heel and lower back are the two areas at highest risk for skin breakdown and formation of bedsores. Several factors make the GBS patient unaware of the risk or unable to take appropriate action. These include confusion or sleepiness, reduced sensation, and paralysis. The first stage of skin breakdown is known as *erythema,* and consists of red or pink discoloration of the skin. The skin over the heels and back *must* be inspected every day for development of erythema. This requires turning the patient onto their side and fully raising the leg so that the possibly affected areas can be properly visualized in good light. Erythema will lead to actual skin breakdown if it is not recognized and aggressively managed. Prevention of skin breakdown is much easier than reversing it once it has developed because infection may occur, making it even more difficult to achieve healing.

Early Occupational and Physical Therapy Care

After initial stabilization in the hospital, occupational and physical therapists should be consulted for evaluation and treatment. During the early days of weakness, the therapists will passively move each joint of each limb through a full range of movement. This will help prevent shortening of the paralyzed muscles *(contractures),* minimize the risk of nerve compression and development of bedsores, and, perhaps just as importantly, it will feel good to the patient. Occasionally, *passive range of motion* exercise is uncomfortable, making it more difficult to persuade the patient of its value. However, the exercises should be continued. In such cases, judicious use of analgesic medications prior to therapy may be useful. In weak patients who are able to move a limb on the bed but not lift it off the bed against gravity, the therapist may assist the movement of the limbs while asking the patient to make an effort. This is referred to as *active assistive range of motion* exercise. Special attention is usually given to the joints of the limbs: the knees, ankles, hips, shoulders, elbows, and wrists. Limb movement may also help maintain an awareness of joint position. Furthermore, the daily presence of a physical and occupational therapist at the bedside provides additional professional monitoring for the development of bedsores. Their presence also acts as a reminder to nurses and other personnel that they should actively participate in the prevention of bedsores.

Many GBS patients develop weakness in the muscles of the ankles and wrists. If the weakness is substantial, footdrop and wristdrop can develop because the patient is too weak to overcome the pull of gravity and keep the feet and hands in a natural, upward position. The downward pull of gravity on the feet can lead to shortening and tightening of the calf tendons and muscles and prevent normal, full movement. Similar problems can occur with the forearm muscles and hand movement. Development of contractures can interfere with the process of rehabilitation. Splinting can be provided to prevent these problems and maintain normal or functional positioning of the joints. This is done by using a stiff supportive device to hold the foot and hand in the desired upward position. Foot and hand splints can be fabricated by the therapists to maintain proper foot and hand positions. For the foot, the usual preferred position is a 90 degrees or at a right angle to the leg; for the hand, the usual position is slightly cocked back, at approximately 20 to 30 degrees to the forearm. Additional methods to prevent footdrop include the use of a footboard attached to the end of the bed, upon which the feet can rest; a "bunny boot," a sheepskin lining cradled in plastic, which enables placement of the foot at a nearly normal angle to the bed; or a Multi-Podus® boot or splint, which cradles the foot and lower leg in soft material and has a cutout at the heel to keep pressure off this area. The Multi-Podus® splint is particularly helpful to patients with poor circulation, such as the elderly and diabetics, to keep pressure off the heels and reduce the risk of heel breakdown.

Rehabilitation is a fundamental part of care for the GBS patient. The goal is to provide interventions early in the disease in order to reduce the risk of late complications.

Variable Rate of Improvement

Once a patient reaches maximal weakness, they may stay at this level for an imperceptibly brief period of time, and then proceed directly into recovery. Alternatively, their maximum weakness may continue for days to weeks before improvement begins. Plans can be made for more intensive rehabilitation once a patient begins to show some improvement. The rate of recovery can vary greatly. Not surprisingly, mildly affected patients make a more rapid and complete recovery. Patients who are severely paralyzed recover slowly and often incompletely. Typically, improvement is more rapid earlier in the recovery phase, and then it slows down. It is important for medical, nursing, and therapy staff to understand that recovery is a slow process. A patient with a slow recovery should never be considered lazy or uncooperative.

CHAPTER 6

Rehabilitation and Coming Home

This chapter provides details of rehabilitative care for the patient with Guillain-Barré syndrome (GBS). Much of this chapter is also applicable to patients with chronic inflammatory demyelinating polyneuropathy (CIDP) and other GBS variants. The main issues covered include the process of deciding upon an optimal rehabilitation setting, the rehabilitation process itself, preparing to go home, and home accommodations for disability.

THE INTERMEDIATE PHASE OF REHABILITATION

Leaving the Acute Care Hospital and Disposition Planning

Most patients start rehabilitation in the acute care hospital. Once the GBS patient is medically stable, planning will begin for the next phase of rehabilitation. The plateau phase of the disease is variable and may last as little as a few days or as long as several weeks, and during this phase the patient does not require the services of an acute care hospital. By this stage, most patients will be able to breathe without assistance, and even if some level of ventilatory support is still needed, the situation will be stable and an intensive care unit (ICU) setting will no longer be necessary. The major role of the acute care hospital for the GBS patient is the treatment of the underlying immunologic disorder with plasmapheresis or intravenous immunoglobulin (see Chapter 7), as well as treatment and stabilization of medical complications of the disorder (see Chapter 5). These activities usually include weaning the patient off the ventilator, stabilizing blood pressure and heart rate, and treating infection and blood clots. Once these goals have been accomplished, some muscle strength has often returned and the patient will be ready for rehabilitation.

Some type of rehabilitation is usually needed for the recovering GBS patient when acute hospital care is no longer necessary. The setting for rehabilitation is determined, in part, by the patient's level of disability and their ability to participate in a therapy program.

There are multiple choices for further rehabilitation:

- *In-patient care in a rehabilitation hospital.* A common requirement to qualify for this intensive rehabilitation setting is the patient's ability to participate in at least 3 hours of therapy a day.

- *Day hospital care.* The patient lives at home and is transported by a wheelchair-accommodating van to the rehabilitation hospital or center for a full day of therapy.
- *Skilled nursing facility.* To qualify for this type of inpatient care, the patient must be able to perform 1 to 3 hours of therapy a day and sleeps at the facility.
- *Out-patient rehabilitation.* This is for the more independent patient who attends an hour or so of therapy during the day, as needed.
- *Home-based therapy.* This is provided by visiting therapists or by following instructions set up by therapists for a home therapy program
- *Nursing home.* These facilities provide low-level rehabilitation, as the patient is able to tolerate. This setting may be appropriate for patients with poor recovery, especially the elderly, who still require assistance for most activities.
- *Extended-or long-term acute care facility.* This type of facility can provide chronic ventilator management, nutritional support, and rehabilitation. This type of facility is indicated for the rare patient who is medically stable but requires protracted mechanical ventilation.

The Decision for In-Patient Rehabilitation

The decision regarding the optimal type and location for rehabilitation will be individualized to each patient's particular needs. Factors taken into account typically include the patient's overall physical condition, strength, endurance, and arm and leg functions, as well as insurance considerations. For example, patients with mild impairment who can walk with assistance of a quad (four-footed) or straight cane (single point) may not need the intense degree of care available in an inpatient rehabilitation facility. They may be able to obtain sufficient care in an outpatient setting. If the patient cannot walk, or requires substantial assistance but is showing slow improvement, transfer to an inpatient rehabilitation hospital setting will usually provide an optimal level of care. Some physicians may be reluctant to place GBS patients in rehabilitation hospitals because of concern about depression. Some patients in rehabilitation hospitals have amputations, strokes, or brain injuries, disorders with limited recovery. Physicians may fear that the GBS patient could become depressed if placed among this population. However, the chance for recovery of the GBS patient is usually good and transfer to a rehabilitation center should be optimistically looked upon as an educational process, an opportunity to relearn the proper use of muscles and to walk again. The possibility of depression should be addressed openly with the patient and the family and the usual excellent outcome should be repeatedly emphasized. The benefits of a stay in a rehabilitation center far exceed the slight risk of depression.

Once a patient in an acute hospital appears to be medically stable and is neurologically improving, disposition plans can be made. Those involved in this planning will include the principal treating physician from the acute care hospital, often a neurologist, the rehabilitation physician (physiatrist), physical and occupational therapists, a nurse who has been involved in the daily acute hospital care, a social worker, and a case manager. If the patient still requires mechanical ventilation, a pulmonologist and a respiratory therapist will also be involved. Typically, insurance coverage will be factored into disposition planning. Most GBS patients will be transferred to an acute rehabilitation hospital where they will receive intensive, daily therapy as an inpatient. One criterion for admission into a rehabilitation hospital is the ability to perform at least 3 hours of therapy daily. If a patient does not have sufficient strength and endurance to participate in 3 hours of therapy, a less intensive level of rehabilitation, in a transitional care unit, skilled nursing facility, personal care facility, or nursing/rehabilitation center may be preferable.

Acute In-Patient Rehabilitation for the GBS Patient

Goal of Rehabilitation

The goal of rehabilitation is to maximize recovery of neuromuscular function and ultimately return to pre-GBS life. Rehabilitation does not hasten nerve healing; it does optimize function of muscles, limbs, and the body in general as the nerves heal. An initial step in the rehabilitation process is a comprehensive systematic assessment of nerve and muscle functions as well as medical, social, and vocational background. This baseline information helps the physicians and therapists to design a customized program that will hopefully enable patients to return to their former life style. Most GBS patients will eventually be able to lead a normal or near-normal life. For those patients with incomplete recovery, the goal is to adapt their lifestyle to persisting functional limitations.

A Team Approach

Rehabilitation is provided by a coordinated team of professionals. Depending upon the patient's needs, the team may include a physiatrist or rehabilitation neurologist (who usually leads the overall care), physical therapist, occupational therapist, nurse, internist, psychologist, and social worker with each team member contributing their particular expertise. The team usually meets at a weekly conference to assess the patient's status, determine progress, and plan further care.

The following description provides the highlights of a "typical" rehabilitation program. Details of individual patient care will vary. Care by physical and occupational therapists may overlap to some degree. The physical therapy (PT) program usually concentrates on an exercise regimen to transition the patient to independent walking. The occupation therapy (OT) program will concentrate on teaching the patient how to best use their regained strength for everyday activities and employment. Some parts of the therapy program detailed below will utilize the skills of both disciplines.

Rehabilitation is accomplished with the coordinated efforts of a team of professionals in order to optimize the patient's care and recovery.

Initial Care in the Rehabilitation Hospital

Upon admission to a rehabilitation hospital, several events will occur. The patient or a family member will supply contact information and basic demographic information in order to verify insurance coverage. A nurse will perform an initial evaluation, including a review of medications and dosing (as provided by the referring hospital), obtain essential information about drug allergies and food preferences (e.g., vegetarian, diabetic), and do a basic physical examination. The attending physician, who is ultimately responsible for the patient's care, will usually be a rehabilitation specialist, a physiatrist. This doctor will review the patient's recent and pre-GBS medical history as well as the transfer medications and other orders (such as heel bootie protectors, catheter care, feeding tube care, and tracheostomy), and will perform a general medical and comprehensive functional neuromuscular examination. This information will guide the doctor in determining which of the transfer orders should be continued and which may need modification. An evaluation of the patient's pre-illness life style will also be assessed as a guide toward setting goals of the rehabilitation program. The patient's pre-GBS life and current medical status will help the physicians determine the need for various therapies (e.g., OT, PT). Therapists in these disciplines will evaluate the patient and develop a plan of care. Elements of the patient's pre-GBS life that will help guide creation of a rehabilitation process include the following:

Vocation

Did the patient lead a sedentary life style; for example, drive to a secretarial job that required a lot of typing but only occasional walking? Was the patient active; for example, worked as a construction worker and carried heavy tools and materials up a ladder? Was the patient's life style something in between; for example, was the patient a traveling salesman who walked only short distances but had to get in and out of the car frequently?

Living Situation

Does the patient live in a one-or two-story house? What is the degree of accessibility for wheelchair or walker use? How many steps are there from the sidewalk into the house? What type of floor coverings are in the house? For example, are there mostly hardwood floors with roomsized rugs that can be easily rolled out of the way to allow for easy wheelchair use, or are most floors carpeted? If the patient lives in a twostory house, is there a bathroom with a sink and commode on the lower floor that will make it possible to live on one level?

Life Style/Leisure Activities

Did the patient participate in sports and other vigorous physical activities, or was the patient's pre-GBS life style largely sedentary?

Relapse in GBS

GBS is a monophasic illness in the great majority of patients; that is, once recovery begins it continues without subsequent deterioration. The most common cause of a setback in the rehabilitation setting is extreme fatigue from overwork or nonspecific deterioration as a result of a urinary tract infection or pneumonia, or possibly blood clots (pulmonary embolism). Rarely, a true GBS relapse occurs, particularly if the patient is transferred to rehabilitation too early in the recovery phase. Deterioration due to overwork will seldom last for more than a few hours; the patient will return to baseline state after a period of rest. Deterioration due to a concurrent illness, such as infection or pulmonary embolism, will last longer, usually until the underlying disorder is identified and effectively treated. If a patient in the rehabilitation setting begins to deteriorate, the possibility of an associated illness should be the first consideration, leading to careful clinical assessment, blood and urine tests, and possibly a chest x-ray. If no concurrent illness is identified, and the deterioration is not relieved by a period of rest and a reduction in physical activity, the possibility of a true GBS relapse should be considered. Readmission to an acute care hospital may be necessary. Fortunately, a true relapse is seldom as severe as the initial illness, although it may still have a major impact on a weak patient. Relapses may respond promptly to the same treatment that was used initially.

An initial evaluation assesses current status and helps physicians and therapists develop a program of care that meets the patient's needs.

In addition to rehabilitation, ongoing care of the patient's pre-GBS medical issues as well as complications of GBS will be provided. Examples include medications for high blood pressure, antibiotics for infections, and anticoagulants for blood clots. Additional physicians may be needed to provide concurrent medical care, such as an internist, pulmonary physician, and neurologist. Psychological evaluation, social service assessment, speech, and recreational therapy consultations may also be provided.

GENERAL FEATURES OF A REHABILITATION PROGRAM

Physical and Occupational Therapy

Patient Goals

It is important to set realistic goals during rehabilitation, both with respect to ultimate recovery and duration of the recovery process. For example, if a GBS patient is still in a wheelchair 6 months after the onset of illness, and their goal is to return to their prior recreational activity of cross-country skiing, the therapist may question the level of the patient's understanding of the disorder and recommend further education. Fortunately, most GBS patients eventually regain all or most of their preillness physical abilities and can return to many of their prior activities.

Initial Therapy Evaluation

As noted above, physical and occupational therapists play a key role in the rehabilitation process. Typically, the initial emphasis in rehabilitation is on regaining mobility, first at the bed level, then in a wheelchair, and finally standing and walking. The physical therapist may supply the majority of care for these activities. In GBS, upper limb strength typically returns before lower limb strength. Thus, early on in the rehabilitation process the occupational therapist starts to retrain patients in the use of their arms and hands, to regain independence in activities of daily living such as hygiene, dressing, eating, and bathing.

The physical therapist may start the program with exercises to maintain tone and strengthen the lower limbs, ultimately leading to independent walking. The initial PT and OT evaluations will usually include an assessment of joint mobility, strength of different muscle group actions (e.g., arm elevation, foot-lowering against resistance), and body movement or mobility in various positions (e.g., on a mat, ability to stand, movements while standing). The therapists will also help the patient to learn to manage fatigue.

Evaluation of Range of Motion of Joints

One of the first assessments is evaluation of joint mobility or range of motion. This will help identify any tendon shortening and muscle contractures that may have developed so an exercise program can be customized to address these problems. The lower and upper limbs will be examined with the patient sitting, if possible, or lying down if sitting is not possible. The range of movement of the limb is assessed at each joint to determine if it can be moved freely through its normal range of motion. This is first done passively, with the patient completely relaxed and the therapist doing all the work (passive range of motion).

In some patients, for example, those with arthritis, some joints may have a limited range of motion that is unrelated to GBS. This initial assessment provides the therapist with realistic goals about how far a patient's therapy can be taken. Next, the therapist has the patient move the joints as much as possible without assistance. This active range of motion uses the patient's own muscle strength to move the limbs. After periods of inactivity, passive and active ranges of movement may be reduced due to stiffness in the capsule around the joints and shortening of the muscles and tendons (contractures). In some cases, these contractures significantly interfere with function. For example, if the Achilles tendon behind the ankle is shortened, the patient may not be able to raise their foot up at the ankle and thus may not be able to walk except on their toes. Similarly, if the fingers are curled into a clawed position because of shortening of the tendons in the forearms and stiffening of the joint capsule in the fingers, the patient may not be able to effectively grip and manipulate buttons and zippers, and may not be able to dress themselves or use the toilet independently. These issues are often identified and treated by the occupational therapist.

One of the most important early components of rehabilitation is increasing the range of movement around joints in preparation for strengthening exercises. If physical and occupational therapy has been meticulous in the acute hospital setting, joint contractures will be minimal and strengthening can begin immediately. If not, an arduous and sometimes painful process of stretching the muscles, tendons, ligaments, and joint capsules must be embarked on before strengthening can take place. In the occasional patient who develops significant contractures, early employment of continuous passive range of motion machines will supply slow constant tension to tendons and muscles around a joint to gently stretch the tissues and alleviate shortening. These may be utilized early on in the acute care hospital and continued in the acute rehabilitation setting. Several machines that are designed for use at specific joints are available. Even if there is full or nearly full range of movement, stretching should be done as part of every exercise program. This will be much easier if there are no contractures. Stretching should be performed very carefully to prevent injury—the goal is to increase the range of movement a small amount each day, not necessarily get back to full suppleness immediately.

Muscle Strength Tests

Testing of muscle strength will be done to obtain baseline information about the patient's current status. For example, the patient will be asked to raise each knee while in the sitting position. The therapist will determine whether the patient can do this, and if so, whether the knees can be held up against the downward pressure of the therapist's hands. Can the arms be moved off the bed, raised up to shoulder level, and straight above the head? Can the hands be moved at the wrists? The degree of muscle strength can be recorded using a standardized grading system as illustrated in Table 6-1. This provides a numerical measure of strength that can be compared from week to week during the rehabilitation process to gauge improvement or deterioration.

Tests of Mobility

In addition to determining baseline joint range of motion and muscle group strength, balance and functional mobility status will also be determined with a series of examinations:

Table 6-1. Medical Research Council Grading

Grade 5	Normal strength.
Grade 4	Patient is able to move a limb against gravity plus some resistance applied by the examiner, but the strength is not normal. For example, the patient can, while sitting, lift the knee up and resist some downward pressure from the examining therapist, but
Grade 3	Patient is able to move a limb against gravity but not against any additional resistance or pressure. For example, from the sitting position, the patient can lift the knee but cannot resist any pressure from the examiner's hand.
Grade 2	The patient is unable to lift against gravity but if gravity is eliminated, the limb can be moved. For example, the patient cannot bend the elbow when the arm is held straight out in front of the body, but when the arm is passively lifted up so that it is

Grade 1	A flicker of muscle contraction can be seen or felt by the examiner, but no movement of the limb occurs.
Grade 0	No evidence of muscle contraction can be discerned by the examiner.

1. *Bed mobility or rolling:* Can the patient roll over in bed? This indicates strength and coordination of the muscles of the back, shoulders, elbows, hips, and knees. It also assesses bedsore risk because a patient who cannot roll over in bed is at greater risk for skin breakdown.
2. *Transfers:* Can the patient transfer from the wheelchair to the bed and vice versa, with or without a sliding board?
3. *Sitting:* Can the patient sit upright (static sitting balance)? Can the patient maintain a sitting position and not fall over if gently pushed to one side, the front, or the back (dynamic sitting balance)?
4. *Wheelchair mobility:* Can the patient use a wheelchair independently, or do they lack sufficient arm strength or grip to do this?
5. *Standing:* Can the patient stand without support (static standing balance)? Can the patient stand with support? Can the patient remain standing without losing their balance when gently but firmly pushed to one side, the front, or the back (dynamic standing balance)?

Typically, GBS patients entering a rehabilitation hospital have already regained enough strength to sit up, but dynamic sitting balance may be diminished. They may not yet be able to stand independently, if at all.

Once baseline strength and functional status have been determined and recorded, the physicians and therapists will design a program to improve strength and function. This will, hopefully, bring the patient from their current level of disability to full activity. Such a program is described below. As the patient proceeds through the rehabilitation program, various types of exercises will be employed. All care is customized to the individual patient's status and goals.

The initial physical and occupational therapy evaluations provide a baseline from which to start an exercise program that is tailored to the individual needs of each patient, according to the degree of their strength and balance.

Types of Exercises

Exercises cannot be performed unless the patient can at least move a limb with gravity eliminated; that is, with at least Grade 2 strength (see Table 6-1). Therapy for any muscle with less than this amount of weakness will simply consist of passive range of motion performed by the therapist. Once Grade 2 is reached, a variety of exercises can be performed with the limb moving parallel to the floor with gravity taken out of play. When the patient reaches Grade 3 strength, it is time to graduate to low-resistance exercises, against gravity and minimal resistance.

Low-Resistance Exercise. The primary goal of *low-resistance* exercise is to increase stamina rather than strength. The patient will do many repetitions of an exercise against minimal resistance rather than a few exercises against greater resistance. Neuromuscular fatigue is a big part of GBS, and GBS patients should only exercise until they begin to sense fatigue. Repetitions with low weight or resistance will improve muscle endurance and fatigue resistance, and increase oxidative muscle capacity. This is known as *aerobic training.* As strength and stamina improve, patients will be asked to do progressively harder exercises, called *highresistance* exercises.

Initial therapy may consist of passive stretching, followed by exercises against low resistance to build up endurance. Fatigue is common in recovering GBS patients, and strength and stamina should be increased slowly.

Muscle-Strengthening/High-Resistance Exercises. In contrast to lowresistance exercises, the primary goal of high-resistance exercise is to increase strength rather than stamina. Of course, both forms of exercise increase strength and stamina, but the primary goals are different. As strength returns, heavier weights can be used with fewer repetitions.

Progressive-Resistance Exercises. As strength further improves, exercises may be added to maximize muscle contraction through the entire range of motion. Machines designed to perform progressive-resistance exercises can be used to accomplish this, with the resistance being increased in relation to strength and endurance.

Most exercises are designed to strengthen specific muscle groups and functions, such as leg extension (raising the leg) and forearm flexion (bending the arm at the elbow). Another approach utilizes a combination exercise that incorporates both strong and weak muscles in a movement. A therapist might, for example, engage a patient in a combined activity of simultaneously bending the hip while also bending the foot up and inward. The goal of combining two or more exercises is to help transfer strength from stronger muscles to weaker ones. The potential benefits of this technique, called *proprioceptive neuromuscular facilitation* (PNF), are ultimately limited by the amount of nerve supply to each muscle group participating in the combined activity. PNF helps to maintain range of motion of the exercised joints.

The following therapies may be utilized to treat the GBS patient. Which of these is used depends on functional status when rehabilitation begins.

Pool Therapy. If the patient cannot stand independently, a first step in therapy may be the use of a pool or "water therapy" for weight bearing to provide buoyancy from water.

Water therapy is ideal because it provides both support and resistance. Initially, the extremely weak patient may be fitted with a life jacket, transferred to a submersible stretcher, lowered into a pool, and assisted into a suitable depth of water, where the motions of walking with partial weight bearing can be performed safely. The life jacket and water provide buoyancy, enabling the patient to relearn how to walk, and the warm temperature of the therapeutic pool can relieve muscle pain.

The exercise pool provides buoyancy to support the body, while also providing warmth to soothe aching muscles. It provides severely weak patients with an excellent way to start the rehabilitation process.

Mat Exercises. Once strength begins to return, exercises on a floor mat can be started. Initially, these exercises are performed with the therapist assisting the movement, then against the resistance of gravity, and finally using weights as resistance. Hip abduction strengthening is one example of mat exercise. While lying on their side, the patient slowly raises the upper leg, initially with the therapist supporting part of the weight, then independently against gravity, and finally against increasing resistance provided by weights or springs. This helps to strengthen the hip abduction muscles at the outer aspect of the hip.

The use of a floor mat for exercise provides the patient who cannot yet stand with the ability to perform a variety of exercises that can help strengthen specific muscle groups in preparation for walking.

Building Strength and Endurance. As nerve supply improves, additional exercises can be added to further develop muscle strength. For example, stationary bicycle pedaling may be used, as well as progressive resistive exercises, which are designed to provide the leg with a constant force as the knee travels through its normal range of motion with the patient sitting. This can be done on an exercise machine.

Exercises, including weight lifting, may be used to improve upper limb strength, and eventually allow the patient to transfer independently from a wheelchair to a bed or a regular chair. Sliding boards are often used to assist in this process. A sliding board is a flat piece of wood or plastic, typically about 3/4 inch thick, 10 inches deep, and 2 1/2 feet wide that enables the patient to slide from chair to bed and back without having to stand. Before transferring, make sure that the wheelchair is locked and that the adjacent chair or bed is also firmly fixed so the board will not slip out of position and cause injury.

Measure of Neuromuscular Function. Throughout the course of rehabilitation, the patient will be evaluated from time to time, perhaps weekly or less often, to determine their ability to perform routine tasks. These tests of neuromuscular strength and other functions measure such activities as ability to perform self care (e.g., eating and grooming), stand up without or with assistance, walking, use of stairs, and social interaction. Impaired neuromuscular functions that underlie identified deficiencies, such as inability in raising the arms, will be measured and recorded in a standardized format or table. The impairment will be analyzed and used to modify the rehabilitation program to improve these actions. An example of such an analysis tool is the *Functional Independence Measure or FIM™ Instrument.*

Safety should always come first. The recovering GBS patient often wants to do as much as they can as soon as they can. However, if balance or standing endurance is poor, the patient can fall, causing injury.

Progression to Walking. As leg strength improves, assistive devices may be used to provide balance and support during walking. The patient will usually begin to walk between parallel bars; two railings placed about 2 feet apart at waist height. The patient can use these bars for support when attempting to walk. A wheeled walker can also be used. Unstable patients can roll the walker in front of them to provide support while walking. As balance improves, a standard, non-wheeled walker can be used, with the patient lifting it ahead of the body when walking. The patient then progresses to crutches and eventually to canes. A quad cane, one with four points on the floor, provides greater stability and is usually used first. When the patient has enough balance and strength, a single-point cane may be sufficient. Eventually, independent walking without an assistive device can usually be accomplished.

Substitution

A phenomenon called *substitution* can occur during rehabilitation. This involves a tendency for stronger muscles to be used at the expense of weaker ones. For example, it is natural to use the hip flexors when walking. These are the muscles that raise the leg in order to move the body forward. However, if the nerve supply to this muscle group is poor, and other muscles can be substituted to move the body forward because they have better nerve supply, there is a tendency to use the stronger muscles. For example, a swing gait can be used to aid walking, but it substitutes for a normal gait. A swing gait involves throwing the hip outward to swing it forward, causing a duck-like waddling pattern. This gait is not normal and should be avoided for the long term. If left unaddressed, the patient will end up with a long-term waddling gait that can lead to hip and back pain. If such a gait is observed during rehabilitation, exercises should be employed to strengthen and emphasize the use of the hip flexor muscles in order to develop a more normal gait.

If substitution of stronger for weaker muscles occurs, customized exercises can be performed to help strengthen the weaker muscles.

Exercise Caveats

Avoid Fatigue. Vigorous efforts and longer therapy sessions will not speed recovery. Pushing muscles to the point of fatigue will lead to exhaustion and delay recovery.

Pain with Exercise. Pain may restrict rehabilitation and should be treated aggressively. Treatment options include various medications, heat, massage, and several others as discussed in Chapter 8. Development of pain during rehabilitation may indicate that too much is being demanded of the patient and that a period of rest may be needed.

Pain is common in GBS, but several methods are available to treat it.

Nerve Regeneration

The rehabilitation process does not improve nerve regeneration, and thus does not affect the return of nerve supply to muscles (muscle innervation). Rather, a major goal of rehabilitation is to assist the patient to optimize the use of their muscles as their nerve supply returns, and to adapt their life style to whatever functional limitations they may end up with due to incomplete recovery.

Rehabilitation does not speed up nerve healing, but rather it is used to optimize use of the limbs and other activities as nerves heal and function improves.

Patterns of Strength Return

Strength usually returns in a *descending pattern,* meaning that arm strength returns before hand strength and upper limb strength returns before lower limb strength. Usually the last function to return is the ability to raise the foot at the ankle. Failure of this function to return can lead to long-lasting, occasionally permanent, foot drop and necessitate the use of a brace, such as an ankle-foot orthosis (AFO) as discussed elsewhere. As arm strength returns, patients will be able to feed and dress themselves again, and as leg strength returns, transferring and walking become possible.

Strength usually returns in a descending pattern, meaning that arm strength returns before hand strength and upper limb strength returns before lower limb strength.

Changing Rate of Recovery

Strength tends to return more rapidly during the earlier phase of recovery, and then slowly tapers down, returning more slowly in the latter stages.

Duration of Recovery

Recovery is the most rapid during the first 6 months after onset of GBS, and is generally complete within 2 to 3 years. However, many patients have described continued, minor improvement long after that period is over. For example, one right handed patient experienced sporadic numbness and tingling of the fifth finger of his right hand for about 6 years, but this eventually stopped. In addition, for about 15 years, to keep his right hand steady he had to anchor his right wrist against a desk and using his left hand to stabilize the right hand. With the right hand anchored he could create smooth curving lines. Eventually he was able to write without bracing the wrist.

Most recovery from GBS occurs within 2 to 3 years, but many patients report small improvements for much longer periods.

Fatigue

Fatigue has important implications for GBS patients in the rehabilitation setting and in general. In many rehabilitation settings, patients are strongly encouraged to exercise to maximal tolerance—the "no pain, no gain" philosophy. However, this is definitely *not* advised for the GBS patient. Excessive exercise can lead to aches, cramps, pain, weakness, and exhaustion of muscles that have inadequate nerve supply. Excessive exercise may lead to a temporary setback. Therefore, moderation or pacing of exercise is advised. Patients generally should be allowed to exercise up to a sense of impending muscle ache and fatigue, but no further. GBS patients are often so determined to get back to normal life that they push themselves too much in an attempt to recover faster, but this leads to exhaustion that will set them back. The astute therapist will recognize the overly zealous patient who pushes too hard, and direct them to rest when fatigue begins to set in.

Fatigue is common in GBS, and exercise should be stopped until after the fatigue has passed.

Emotional Reactions

Strong emotional reactions to GBS are normal, and the rehabilitation unit may be a place of great emotional outpouring, including euphoria when independence in even the simplest tasks is achieved. Most GBS patients show progressive improvement during the rehabilitation process. Remember, GBS is *monophasic,* meaning it usually happens only once. After reaching the point of the most severe weakness, the usual pattern is continued improvement. It may be slow, but each improvement in the ability to perform routine tasks will be considered a great accomplishment.

Assistive Devices

During rehabilitation, emphasis is placed on proper body mechanics, avoidance of substitution of stronger muscles for weaker ones, and prevention of muscle strain and fatigue. For patients with persisting muscle group weakness, assistive devices (orthotics) can be used to circumvent disability. For example, a dropped foot can be treated with a *molded ankle-foot orthosis* (MAFO). This is

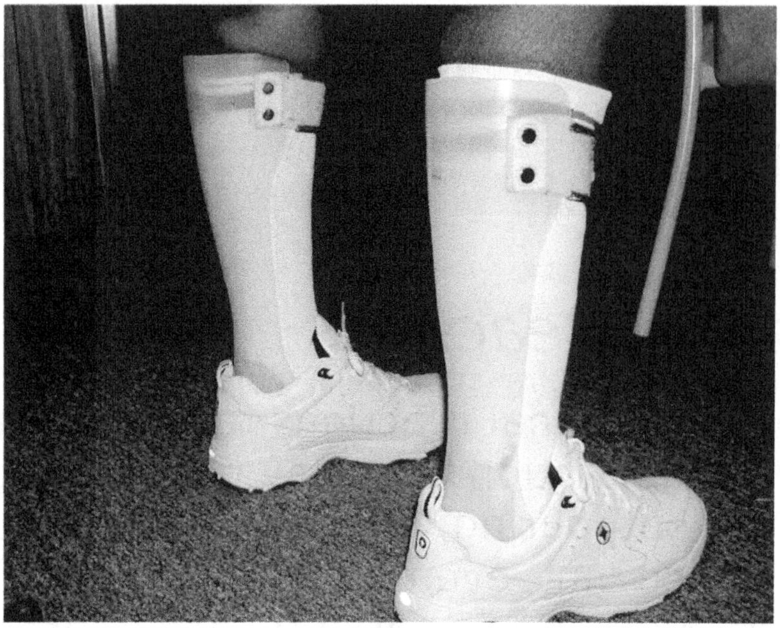

FIGURE 6-1: Molded ankle foot orthosis (MAFO).

a lightweight, plastic device that wraps behind the leg and under the foot. As depicted in Figure 6-1, the MAFO is made of thin, white plastic. It is hardly noticeable when the pant legs are down. The person in this figure is wearing a high, thick sock that provides a soft cushion between the firm plastic splint and the skin. The thin, plastic material often allows the patient to wear regular shoes rather than getting larger ones. Depending upon the patient's gait abnormality, the MAFO may have a fixed angle between the leg and foot or be hinged with spring loading. The hinge may incorporate adjustable stops in order to limit the amount of upward foot movement *(dorsiflexion)* and downward movement *(plantar flexion)* during walking. The goal is to stabilize the ankle and foot, and assure that the forefoot can be raised sufficiently to gain enough toe clearance to avoid tripping.

Some patients may experience persisting difficulty in the use of their hands and fingers when performing such activities as fastening clothing, writing, using utensils, and handling objects. Methods to compensate for these problems are available. For example, a button-hooking device may be used to circumvent difficulty in buttoning clothes. Velcro® straps or zippers with large pull handles may sometimes be a practical alternative to buttons. Severely affected patients are taught ways to conserve energy by using shortcuts to maximize hand and arm use. Splints may be used to position the wrist slightly cocked and to support the thumb in order to restore maximum use of the hand.

For the patient with a weak grip, utensil handles can be fitted with a thick barrel of foam rubber to enable better gripping of the utensil. The edge of a plate can be fitted with a raised metal rim so the patient can push food against it with a fork or spoon in order to get the food onto the utensil. A Velcro® strap can be placed around a cane handle to help a patient with a poor grip hold onto the handle, allowing use of the cane.

Simple assistive devices can be very helpful. A thick-handled fork may enable a patient with a poor grip to be able to eat independently. Usually the need for such devices is temporary.

Activities of Daily Living

Activities of daily living (ADL) is a cover phrase for some of the essential activities of every day life, such as hygiene care, eating, dressing, writing, and vocational activities. Relearning these basic activities is an important part of rehabilitation for the GBS patient. Instructing and guiding the patient to perform ADL typically falls under the domain of the occupational therapist since they concentrate on exercises to regain upper limb function. As with the lower limbs, function of the upper limbs usually returns in a proximal to distal pattern. Thus, use of the shoulders, that part of the upper limb closer, or more proximal to the central part of the body, will typically return before use of the hands and fingers, those parts of the upper limb further from the center of the body. During rehabilitation, testing of neuromuscular strength will be performed on a regular basis, every week or so, to identify weak muscle function. The therapy program will be adjusted to direct strengthening exercises to these muscle groups. If, for example, grip strength is weak, the patient may be provided with a rubber ball to squeeze repeatedly in order to strengthen the flexion muscles of the hand and fingers that form the grip. To strengthen the muscles of the fingers, a rubber band may be placed across the fingers, and the patient instructed to alternately spread the fingers apart and then bring them back together. The force of the rubber band against the spreading fingers provides resistance for finger movement.

Tests may be used to determine the amount of sensation in the hands. For example, the patient may be instructed to look away while placing a hand into a bowl of sand containing articles of varied consistency and shape, such as a marble, key, eraser, pen, and closed safety pin. The ability of the patient to identify the objects in the container of sand (without looking at them) from their particular shape and consistency provides a measure of how much sensation has returned to the hands. If adequate function or use does not return to the hands, various assistive devices, as described above, can be employed.

As part of the ADL experience and transitioning the patient for returning to home, a *model apartment* in the rehabilitation hospital may be used, as described below, in the "Preparing to Go Home" section.

In addition to the contributions by occupational and physical therapists as described above, other therapists make important contributions to the patient's care as outlined in the section below on page 134, "Transition to Home and Planning for the Future" and in Chapter 8.

Other Components of the Rehabilitation Process

Physical and occupational therapists supply most of the physical rehabilitation for the GBS patient, but additional care may also involve a recreational therapist, rehabilitation nurse, social worker, psychologist, and psychiatrist.

Recreational Therapy

Recreational therapy can have particular value for the patient with ongoing disability. Engagement in recreational activities helps accustom the patient to participation in leisure events within the limits of their disability. Most importantly, this type of therapy helps incorporate the reality that their disability is a part of them, but they can still enjoy life. Recreational therapy may involve all levels of activities, including watching television as part of a group, playing bingo, and wheelchair basketball.

Speech Therapy

Speech therapists are often as involved in the evaluation of swallowing as they are in helping to improve enunciation. They really should be called *speech/swallowing therapists.* Both of these functions involve the use of nerves and muscles that can be affected in GBS.

Speech and swallowing are occasionally affected in GBS. In severe cases, the patient on a respirator will be unable to speak because the tube placed into the airway does not allow movement of the vocal cords, which normally produce sound. These patients can usually communicate via Communication Cards (see Chapter 2). Typically, after an endotracheal tube is removed, the patient's speech returns within a few days. Even without prior use of a respirator, a patient may still find talking difficult if the muscles used for speech have been weak. These muscles include those of the vocal cords, tongue, lips, and mouth. Slurred speech or difficulty swallowing may occur. A speech therapist can help the patient learn exercises for the affected muscles in order to improve speech patterns and clarity of the voice, as well as recommend dietary changes to facilitate safe swallowing with adequate nutrition.

Patients who were on a respirator for more than 2 weeks will likely have had a tracheostomy tube inserted through a hole in the front of their neck. Once the tube is removed, they may require additional help in speaking clearly until the hole closes completely. A patient who has had a protracted stay in the ICU may require reeducation about safe swallowing and clear speech.

Psychologists and Psychiatrists

These therapists can play an important role in assisting patients and families in dealing with the new and sometimes overwhelming problems of paralysis, dependency, loss of income, and a multitude of associated emotional problems. Emotional reactions to severe illness can include frustration, depression, self-pity, denial, anger, and fear. In spite of the potential gravity of the illness, the prognosis for the GBS patient is optimistic. Therefore, a practical approach is to take one day at a time during the rehabilitation process, with an attitude of cautious optimism. The psychologist can guide patients and families in dealing with the emotional impact of illness. The psychologist may use talk therapy to help them understand that their fear, anger, and other emotions are common and understandable, and that they should not feel guilty about their feelings. Validating the legitimacy of the emotional reactions to GBS, and offering a supportive, understanding ear can help ease fear and lead patients and their families to acceptance. The goal is to help GBS patients and their families deal with whatever physical limitations may persist in a constructive manner.

Psychiatrists are medical doctors licensed to prescribe medications. The psychiatrist will evaluate the patient's emotional status, correlate it with their personality, and then provide medications, such as antidepressants, to ease the patient's stress and improve their ability to cope. The psychiatrist, psychologist, social worker, and other therapists will analyze the patient's attitude toward their illness in order to determine if the patient is being realistic. If not, they will try to guide the patient toward a more realistic outlook. This is often done with talk therapy, to provide reinforcement to the patient about their medical and rehabilitation status, prognosis, and plan of care.

GBS is stressful to both patients and their loved ones. It is natural to be scared and even overwhelmed by worries about the future. Guidance from professionals should be welcomed.

Rehabilitation Nurses

Rehabilitation nurses are central players in recovery from GBS. They see the patient more often than any other member of the team. Their duties are myriad; they dispense medications, assist with bathing, deal with catheters, provide emotional support, meet family members and other visitors, and act as a liaison between the physicians and various therapists. They give the most hands-on care. They may be the first one to recognize when the patient has a medical complication or emotional problem. They will also be the ones visitors ask for information about the patient's status.

Social Workers

From day one of a GBS patient's care in the acute care hospital and thereafter, a social worker will usually be involved. They serve many roles. At the acute care and rehabilitation hospitals, they will document the patient's insurance coverage and review the home environment and employment with the patient and their immediate family. They will monitor the patient's progress, so that when discharge from a facility is contemplated, they will have sufficient information with which to plan for a suitable place for the patient to go. The goal is to prepare the patient, within the limits of their illness, to be discharged to the next most appropriate facility. For the patient in the acute care facility, who is safely out of the ICU, the next step is usually a rehabilitation hospital, and then home.

Fortunately, most GBS patients can look forward to a full recovery, and the rehabilitation process is designed to help them recover. However, in this era of limited resources and restrictive insurance policies, it is not uncommon for patients to be discharged from the rehabilitation hospital before they are fully recovered. This is especially true if they have reached a plateau in their rehabilitation process, or if they have sufficient strength and accommodations so that they can be safely discharged to their home. An occasional patient, particularly the elderly, may not have sufficient strength even when they reach maximum improvement to manage at home, and they may be need to be placed in an assisted living or personal care community. The social worker will evaluate the patient's overall situation, including their ability to move around and attend to the normal activities of daily life, the physical and mental abilities of their caregivers, and the safety of the home environment, in order to help the patient and the family reach a decision as to the next step.

The social worker will access the patient's abilities as discharge time approaches so they can be referred to an appropriate living situation. Most patients can eventually return home.

Rehabilitation therapists will often provide additional care after the patient is discharged from the acute care and/or rehabilitation hospital. Specifics of further outpatient therapy needs and care are described below and in Chapter 8 in the section, *The Severely Disabled Patient at Home.*

TRANSITION TO HOME AND PLANNING FOR THE FUTURE

Preparing to go home represents a major transition in the recovery process. After discharge from inpatient rehabilitation, patients will usually continue therapy in some type of outpatient program. Eventually the patient will reach a level of maximum improvement, and formal rehabilitation will be over. How is this decision made? The answer is quite practical. Typically, the patient's physical and occupational therapists will record the patient's abilities on a regular basis and report their findings to the physiatrist. Most patients will continue to improve until they can walk independently. An occasional patient will reach maximum improvement or plateau before this point. The therapists will monitor the patient to look for evidence of either continued improvement or a plateau. One example of reaching a plateau, short of full recovery, is the ability to stand up and walk with a walker but *not* have the ability to use a crutch or cane.

Typically, if a patient shows lack of improvement over about 3 weeks, they may have reached a plateau. This does not mean there will be no further improvement, but it may signal the need for less intensive therapy. If the plateau falls short of independent walking, long-term living accommodations will need to be arranged.

A major goal of rehabilitation is the ability to walk independently. Most GBS patients will reach this goal. Once it is reached, the patient may or may not also be completely back to normal. It is common for the GBS patient, who can now walk independently, to still experience some weakness, fatigue, and abnormal sensations, such as tingling and pain.

> Most GBS patients regain the ability to walk independently. However, some of them may still experience abnormal sensations and/or fatigue.

These remaining symptoms may warrant further rehabilitation and medical attention.

Preparing to Go Home

Returning home involves much preparation. Criteria for discharge to home will take into account several variables. What is the insurance coverage? If the patient is still using a wheelchair, but is good at transfers from wheelchair to bed and back, is there good access to the house? Is the entrance ramped? Does the patient live in an elevator building? Can the patient safely live on one floor with the help of supportive, capable caregivers? Discharge to home with day hospital care may be an excellent option if these criteria are in place. Patients who participate in day hospital care have breakfast at home, are picked up by a van that can accommodate wheelchairs, and are driven to the hospital for a full day of therapy. At the end of the day, they are transported by van back home to have dinner and sleep. Alternatively, home-based care using a visiting nurse, physical therapist, and occupational therapist may be used.

The home will need to be evaluated to make sure it can accommodate the patient's current level of ability and disability. Is there a firstfloor bathroom or a commode? Is there a private place to sleep on the first floor? Is the house or apartment accessible by wheelchair, either by ramp or elevator? Remember, even one step will make the next level inaccessible to a wheelchair unless it is ramped.

Typically, the rehabilitation hospital will designate a registered nurse or social worker from a home-care company to meet with the family and plan for the patient's return to home. Together, they will determine if the transfer is realistic and safe.

The Model Apartment

One method in planning for discharge to home with accommodation to the patient's ADL needs is a trial overnight stay in a model apartment in the acute rehabilitation hospital. This apartment usually has a bedroom, bathroom, and eat-in kitchen. In this trial setting, the patient will go through the actual process of preparing for bed, with night time hygiene, changing of clothes, and getting into bed. In the morning, the patient will arise, bathe, dress, prepare a meal, and wash dishes. These seemingly simple tasks, may, for the recovering GBS patient, present many challenges. The monitoring of the patient's activities in this setting by the rehabilitation team will often help identify issues that warrant accommodation at home, from large handled utensils for gripping, to a higher toilet seat with side rails, to grab bars at pertinent places, etc. These issues are discussed in some detail below.

In all aspects of the patient's life, their caregivers will likely be helping out more when the patient initially returns home, and less as the patient's strength and endurance return. Some accommodations that may be warranted include:

Entrance Modifications

The entrance to the living quarters can be modified to accommodate the limitations of the recovering GBS patient as follows:

1. *Ramping.* This should be done at an incline of 1 foot of length for each inch of elevation. Thus, in order to rise 8 inches (the height of one step), an 8-foot length of ramp will be needed; 38 inches is a good width. Ramps for long-term use should have a railing on both sides for safety. Safety railings are often required by local regulations. If the ramp will only be needed for a short time and the person pushing the patient is strong enough, a steeper incline may be built using an 8-inch length for each 1 inch of rise.
2. *Good lighting.* Good lighting will help provide an added measure of safety if there is the remotest chance that the ramp will be used in the dark.
3. *Cover from the elements.* Rain and snow can be a real annoyance when trying to handle a wheelchair while searching for keys. A covered, well-lit entrance can be quite helpful in this situation.

Bathroom Modifications and Hygiene

The following modifications can be made to the bathroom for the safety and convenience of the person recovering from GBS:

1. Elevated toilet seat, firmly fixed to the top of the toilet.
2. Bars on both sides of the toilet that the patient can grab and push up on to facilitate transfer; elevated toilet seats often have these bars built in.
3. Seat in the shower and/or grab bars so patients can anchor themselves safely and securely.
4. Hand-held shower within easy reach.
5. Hook from which the patient can take a towel to dry off.
6. Shower *without* a glass door; glass can shatter if broken and cause injury. Glass doors can be lifted off the sliding track, or the hinges removed, and then replaced with a shower curtain.
7. A portable commode will work in place of a toilet if there is no accessible bathroom. The commode will need to be emptied frequently to prevent unpleasant odors. If delay in emptying is anticipated, for example, when a caregiver is going to be absent for a protracted length of time, a toilet deodorant can be used. This liquid (available in marine supply stores), sometimes called "head and holding tank chemical treatment" breaks down waste and provides a pleasant scent.
8. A kitchen or bathroom sink can be used. However, a hand-held wash basin may make more sense if the patient cannot stand upright to use the sink.

9. Wet soap is slippery and can be a real challenge. "Soap on a rope" can be used as an alternative. You can make your own by drilling a hole in a bar of soap, tying a rope through it, and then attaching it to something in a convenient location, such as around the bottom of the cold water handle. (Using the hot water handle risks a burn.) Nylon rope, 1/8 of an inch in diameter, will easily withstand water and heat.
10. An electric shaver will be easier and safer to use than a regular razor until grip strength and dexterity return.
11. A sonic or electric toothbrush can be used if handling a regular toothbrush is too difficult.

Dining

These accommodations will make it easier for the recovering GBS patient to eat:

1. Remove the arms of the wheelchair, if one is used, in order to roll it closer to the table.
2. Sliding onto a regular dining chair from a wheelchair is an option if the patient is able to transfer. An assistant will be needed to move the chairs close together to facilitate the transfer.
3. There are several options if hand and finger use are limited. As discussed in the section on assistive devices, a dinner plate with a high rim can be used to prevent food from falling off the plate as it is pushed onto a spoon or fork. Utensils with thick handles are easier to grip. Occupational

therapists are often aware of companies that sell this type of equipment.

4. Eating can trigger the urge to urinate or defecate, so be prepared.
5. The patient's taste buds may not yet be back to normal. Try to be more imaginative with various spices, and perhaps use the usual ones more liberally. Serve attractive foods that the patient likes, and provide multivitamins or other supplements as recommended by the doctor.

Steps

Trying to climb up even one step while dependent on a walker may seem like trying to climb a mountain to a person recovering from GBS. If the patient cannot yet climb steps, first-floor living with accommodations for disabilities is mandatory. The outdoor ramps described above can also be constructed for use indoors. Steps must be avoided if they cannot be climbed.

Wheelchair Use

Many recovering GBS patients will need to use a wheelchair, although this will be temporary for most of them. Family members and other caregivers need to be patient and loving with the GBS patient and with each other. Everybody's disposition may be stressed by living with someone in a wheelchair, and they may feel like it will go on forever. However, the patient will improve gradually, over time, and eventually the wheelchair can be eliminated.

Always remember: safety first when using a wheelchair. Avoid falls; the landing can be painful and possibly break something. It is far better to take the time to secure the wheelchair. ALWAYS lock the wheels before getting in or out of the wheelchair, and transfer to a secured chair or bed.

Clothing

Changes in clothing may be necessary, and the following may be helpful:

1. Clothes that fit prior to GBS may be too loose if there was some weight loss. Velcro® strips, moving buttons, or a temporary inexpensive wardrobe may be helpful until the patient's normal weight is regained.
2. Zippers typically use small pulls. If grip or dexterity is lacking, a key ring can be put through the end of the zipper pull to supply a larger grip.
3. Patients who were on a ventilator may have a larger neck than they did before they became ill. A button extender can be used to allow closure of the top of a man's shirt. Button extenders can be purchased from The Vermont Country Store (see Resources: Miscellaneous Accommodations).
4. Shoes that fit prior to the GBS may no longer fit. They may be too loose, or more likely too

tight if the patient developed foot swelling from inactivity. If new shoes are needed, here are few suggestions: Do not buy shoes according to size. Instead, buy shoes that are comfortable and attractive to the patient. If one foot is bigger (more swollen) than the other, buy the larger pair so they fit the larger foot comfortably. Inner padding can be used under the shoe tongue to tighten up the loose shoe so it will also fit comfortably. If possible, find shoes with Velcro® straps instead of shoe laces. These can be worn until hand dexterity and general agility return. Of course, slipons and loafers are preferred, as long as they are not so loose that they fall off, possibly causing an accident.

Most GBS patients are not fully independent when they are discharged from inpatient rehabilitation to home. Yet, this transition usually represents a major accomplishment. Advance preparation can help make it a more positive experience.

Medications

Multiple medications can be organized for ease and accurate usage. A large-capacity, plastic pill box may be helpful. Purchase one that has separate places for Sunday through Saturday medications, and a place each day for morning, midday, dinnertime, and bedtime medications. The compartments can also be relabeled to comply with the patient's medication regimen. Fill all the appropriate spaces carefully once a week with the drugs needed for each day. Medications that are "as needed" or "prn" can be kept in separate bottles. Most pharmacies dispense medications in round plastic bottles, and this may create several problems. If the bottle lands on the floor, it could be stepped on and cracked. Store bottles in a safe place, such as a tray with 1+ inch side walls, so they cannot fall on the floor. The round shape of the bottle makes reading the label awkward. Consider using a felt-tipped marker to add labeling so you know what the medicine is and how to use it. Additional labeling can be put on a piece of white adhesive tape and attached to the bottle. Many labels only list the generic name of the drug, which may be difficult to pronounce and unfamiliar to the patient or their family. It may be easier to add trade names to the label. For example, the generic name "diltiazem" can be a tongue twister. Adding the more familiar name Cardizem® might be easier; likewise, Inderal® can be added to the label for propanolol, and Motrin® can be added to the label for ibuprofen.

It is helpful for patients to know what medications they are taking and why, so they can discuss any proposed changes or side effects with their doctors. Most medications are safe, but if discomfort follows the start of a new medication, call the doctor.

Therapy at Home

New issues may arise when the patient comes home. What level of care will the patient require? If therapy at home is planned, who will provide it and how will it be financed? What about making plans to return to work? Financial coverage for care by visiting nurses and therapists is usually covered by the patient's insurance plan. Typically, the nurse and therapists will update the patient's family doctor or other appropriate physician, such as a physiatrist, about any changes in the patient's status, care needs, improvements, or new problems. Any change in care will often be discussed during a telephone call between the therapist and the doctor. Then the therapist will send the doctor a formal, written report for the physician to sign and return to the home-care company. In this manner, all parties are kept informed about the patient's changing status and needs, and the insurance company is supplied with the documentation they need to continue providing medical coverage. If home care is expected to be extensive and involve multiple therapists, a caseworker may be involved; typically a social worker who is familiar with the patient's medical issues and insurance coverage.

If this person represents the insurance company, be aware that their point of view may reflect this.

Returning to Work

A return to work can be planned as the patient's strength and endurance improve. The issues faced in returning to work will depend on the patient's degree of recovery, fatigue, and work demands, both physical and mental.

Vocational accommodations are not that dissimilar to those required at home. Patients need appropriate access to the work site when they return to work. This may include a handicapped parking space near a ramped entrance, a means to get through the entrance doorway (it has to be wide enough for a wheelchair, have a door that can be readily opened, and a relatively flat threshold or floor between outside and inside), and a means to get from the building's entrance level to the work level. For the employee who normally moves around as part of their job, returning to their original employment may not be realistic. For example, the traveling salesman, telephone lineman, or plumber may not be able to return to this type of work if they still require crutches or a wheelchair. Such a situation is rare because most GBS patients eventually improve sufficiently to be able to return to their original work.

Typically, a GBS patient will be able return to work but not until they can walk independently. By then, fatigue is usually not a major problem, and the patient can do some productive work. Of course, this depends on the patient's vocation. As an example, the normal work obligations of the author, a vascular internist, involved walking from his consultation room in his office suite to various examining rooms to see patients. He also would normally go to at least one hospital each day to do hospital rounds on various floors of the hospital. He would normally walk the stairs of the hospital rather than use the elevators. However, as he was recovering from GBS, once he could walk, he did return to work, but at a very limited level. He would be driven to the office by his wife, take the elevator to the second floor, walk about 50 feet to an examining room, see three to four patients over the next hour in that one room, and then either nap or go home to rest. His work required an alert mind, attentive body language, and occasional standing to do an exam, as well as writing. An hour of work was all that was tolerated before fatigue would obligate rest. Over the next weeks and months, he found that he could increase the length of his work day, 1 hour at a time, every several weeks, until eventually he could put in a full day. Six months later, he could sprint briefly, but not walk more than a block or two without becoming exhausted.

Thus, it is readily apparent that each individual patient must accommodate to their own particular disabilities, and this will usually improve with time. A rare patient may experience prolonged substantial disability, and thus require accommodations from the workplace and employer. In this day and age of an unprecedented appreciation to accommodate the disabled, the workplace will hopefully be receptive and able to provide a suitable work environment for the poorly recovered GBS patient.

CAVEATS FOR CAREGIVERS

Emotional Challenges

It is not uncommon for caregivers to experience more emotional conflicts than patients, who may have been preoccupied with trying to get better and following the directions of their doctors and therapists. The healthy family member, who may also be the primary caregiver, may have been trying to handle two sources of stress: visiting and caring for the patient while simultaneously trying to run a household, often raising children and seeing to finances. It can be a harrowing time when the day does not seem long enough to get everything done. It is a time to seek and accept assistance from family, friends, church members, and other resources in your life and community. Let others help with simple day-to-day activities, such as bringing over a prepared dinner, helping with the laundry, or taking a child to a dental appointment.

A Time for Love

Hopefully, by the time the patient returns home, they will be strong enough to be able to use a wheelchair, transfer to a bed, and perhaps even get around with a walker. This will be the case in 50 to 80 percent of patients. Issues in the hospital, such as positioning to avoid bedsores and tender skin that is painful to touch, may no longer be issues by the time the patient is strong enough to return home.

If the patient still has poor use of the hands, some of the basics of self-care, such as shaving, hair washing, and even a haircut or trim, may fall to the responsibility of the main caregiver. Visits from family and friends should be encouraged, but kept short if the patient still tires easily. The patient and their family have been through a frightening experience, and a healthy future may not yet be certain. They will need ongoing encouragement.

Be Patient

Discharge from the hospital and the return home is usually looked upon as a major accomplishment, a time to be thankful. But be aware that there may still be frustrating days and weeks ahead as the patient continues to undergo therapy. Recovery can be slow, and it is best to compare progress by looking at accomplishments week-to-week not day-to-day. The fatigued patient may look fine sitting in a chair, but when they doze off or slump over, understand that their nerves are worn out and their body needs a rest. It takes time for the fatigue of GBS to wane and resolve.

Ongoing Medical Care

Hopefully, a well-orchestrated group of professionals is in place to oversee any continued care that may be needed. This can be set up prior to discharge by the rehabilitation hospital's social service/discharge planning/care management department (the name of the department will vary from hospital to hospital). GBS patients who continue rehabilitation at home typically have a social worker to appraise the family's current and long-term needs, a registered nurse to monitor medication use, physical and occupational therapists to provide hands-on therapy and access the patient's long-term needs if good recovery has not occurred, and a physician to oversee treatment.

Practical Guides to Care

Many small issues may warrant attention. For example, if the patient's senses have been compromised, the caregiver may need to check the bath water to make sure the temperature is safe. Good nutrition should be encouraged, especially if the patient has lost weight. If the patient pushes for more activity than they can safely do, some gentle reminders and even scolding may be in order. For example, there is a risk of dropping things and of burn accidents while cooking if good grip has not returned. The use of a microwave oven will reduce the risk of burns, but it is important to be aware that microwave cooking can make food too hot to be safely handled. Do not remove food from the microwave oven immediately, but wait until it is cool enough to handle and eat.

One of the keys to success in recovery is moderation. This is especially true for the overzealous patient who would like to be able to do more than is reasonable. These situations can readily foster frustration. It may help patients and caregivers to vent their feelings and plan together to get through these rough times with an expectation of slow, steady improvement.

CHAPTER 7

Immunotherapy Treatment

Guillain-Barre syndrome (GBS) is a disease in which the majority of Gpatients will make an excellent functional recovery. It is therefore extremely important that any treatment does no harm. Although some recently introduced treatments accelerate the rate of recovery and may reduce the residual neurologic deficits, the primary goal of treatment is still to provide supportive care during the acute illness so that the natural process of recovery can occur. Because of the substantial risks from respiratory failure and autonomic instability, all patients with GBS, no matter how mild their symptoms may initially appear, should be admitted to a hospital with an intensive care unit (ICU). It is impractical to expect all patients to be admitted to an ICU, but anyone with declining pulmonary function or demonstrated autonomic instability, such as irregular heart rhythm or unstable blood pressure, should be closely monitored in the intensive care setting.

IMMUNOTHERAPY

The evidence that GBS is an autoimmune disease is circumstantial, but overwhelming. Therefore, attempts to reduce the severity of the disease and accelerate recovery have concentrated on manipulation of the immune system with *immunotherapy.* There are two forms of immunotherapy for GBS that have been shown to accelerate recovery: plasma exchange and intravenous immunoglobulin (IVIg). No treatment has been shown to definitely reduce the initial severity of GBS.

The proven effective treatments for GBS are generally safe, but they are not entirely free of risk. As with any disease and any treatment, the severity of the disease and the risk of treatment must be considered when deciding whether to treat. Not all GBS patients need to be treated. As a general guide, if the GBS patient is able to walk without assistance, treatment with immunotherapy may not be necessary. However, there are exceptions to this rule. Occasional patients may still be able to walk but have difficulty breathing or may have compromised swallowing functions. Such patients are at substantial risk and should be treated. Patients with Miller Fisher syndrome (see Chapter 1) generally have an excellent prognosis, and life-threatening complications, such as respiratory failure or aspiration, are rare so treatment is generally not recommended unless balance is severely affected. On the other hand, if there are factors that predict a poor outcome, such as low-amplitude motor responses on electrodiagnostic testing, antecedent diarrhea due to *Campylobacter jejuni* infection or a short interval between the antecedent event and the onset of neurologic symptoms, treatment could be started even if the patient is still able to walk. Similarly, if the progression of the neurologic disability is rapid, treatment could be instituted early.

The most important aspect of GBS treatment is meticulous supportive care, including support of respiration. In those unable to walk, immunotherapy can accelerate recovery. In those still able to walk, treatment decisions should be made on a case by case basis.

PLASMA EXCHANGE (PLEX)

Plasma exchange (PLEX) is a technique that separates the red and white blood cells from the plasma using a special machine. A large needle is inserted into a vein—usually in the arm but sometimes one of the larger veins in the neck—and blood is withdrawn in the same way that it would be withdrawn for a blood donation. The blood is passed into the PLEX machine, which separates the cells from the fluid (plasma). The plasma is discarded and the blood cells are returned to the body, along with an albumin solution from a donor. A single PLEX takes 2 to 3 hours, rarely longer, depending on tolerability, and is typically repeated five times. PLEX is a low-risk procedure. There may be problems associated with catheter placement such as bleeding and infection and there is a small risk of low blood pressure (hypotension) during the treatment and occasional allergic reactions to the replacement fluid. The risks of PLEX are minimized by treatment at a center experienced with the procedure. PLEX should be used with caution in patients who already have documented autonomic instability, such as rapid or irregular heartbeat or fluctuating blood pressure, as it may make this worse. PLEX can also cause anemia, but this is generally mild and does not need treatment.

Why does such a strange procedure help GBS patients? The plasma is presumed to contain the antibodies that cause the demyelination of peripheral nerves. Removing the antibodies presumably allows the nerves to reconstitute the myelin sheaths more rapidly, leading to a quicker recovery.

The use of PLEX in GBS was first reported in 1978. Early uncontrolled reports were euphoric, but not all studies showed a benefit. Because of these conflicting early reports, a multicenter trial of PLEX in North America was started in 1980, and the results were reported in 1985. This was a large study; 122 patients were treated with plasmapheresis, and 123 received conventional, supportive treatment. Patients were randomly assigned to the two groups and all patients were treated within 4 weeks of the onset of weakness. All of these patients had severe weakness; they were unable to walk more than a few steps without assistance. Treatment was administered over 7 to 14 days. Patients who were treated with PLEX improved more rapidly, required ventilator assistance for shorter periods of time, and spent less time in intensive care units and less overall time in the hospital. There was no difference between PLEX and conventional supportive care in terms of mortality or relapses of GBS. The benefit was seen at 4 weeks and at 6 months after the onset of symptoms. PLEX was most beneficial when started early, within a week of the onset of symptoms. There was less benefit if treatment was started more than 2 weeks after onset of symptoms. Patients with low motor amplitudes on electrodiagnostic testing, presumably reflecting a greater degree of axonal degeneration, consistently fared worse than those with normal motor responses, but PLEX also improved the prognosis in that subgroup of patients. A similar French study, published in 1987, confirmed these results.

PLEX is a safe and effective treatment for severe GBS that can be used in all age groups. It accelerates the rate of recovery, but does not reduce mortality or improve the ultimate degree of recovery.

Very few children were included in either of the major controlled studies. In the French study, patients had to be at least 16 years of age, and in the North American study, at least 12 years of age. However, some uncontrolled studies have reported that PLEX is both safe and effective in children even as young as 11 months old.

INTRAVENOUS IMMUNOGLOBULIN (IVIG)

Human plasma (blood with the cells removed) contains proteins called *immunoglobulins.* These immunoglobulins can be separated from the rest of the plasma and a concentrated solution administered intravenously (intravenous immunoglobulin, or IVIg). In GBS, IVIg is administered through a needle or a plastic cannula that is inserted into a vein, usually in the arm. Unlike PLEX, it is rarely necessary to administer the drug into the large neck veins. IVIg is typically administered every day for 5 consecutive days.

IVIg is obtained from donated blood, and contains all of the antibodies of the donor blood. It seems paradoxical to administer antibodies to a patient who is experiencing a disease that results from antibodies attacking the nerves. The exact mechanism of action of IVIg in GBS is not known. One theory is that nonspecific antibodies in the donor IVIg might bind to the specific antimyelin antibodies attacking the nerves in GBS patients and neutralize them. Regardless of the mechanism, IVIg has been shown to be effective in a wide range of autoimmune diseases, including GBS and chronic inflammatory demyelinating polyneuropathy (CIDP).

In a study from the Netherlands, GBS patients were treated with either IVIg or PLEX within 2 weeks of disease onset. Patients receiving IVIg fared better in almost all respects. The time to recovery of walking was 14 days less for patients treated with IVIg, and the time on a ventilator for those with respiratory failure was 7 days less. IVIg also seemed to reduce the severity of weakness, perhaps because treatment was started early (an average of 6 days after onset off the first symptom). Almost twice as many of the patients treated with PLEX required assisted ventilation. These differences in intensive care unit and hospital stay translate into enormous savings in overall health care, as well as benefit to the patient's physical and emotional health. IVIg was also better tolerated than PLEX. Complications of PLEX were almost twice as common as those of IVIg and tended to be more serious. Sixteen percent of the patients treated with PLEX had to have one or more courses stopped because of complications, whereas none of the IVIg patients had significant adverse effects. Other advantages of IVIg are that it is easier to administer, needs no special equipment, and requires a shorter treatment period.

IVIg is not totally risk free and should not be used without serious consideration. The most common problem with IVIg is an allergic reaction to the protein contained in the product. This is usually mild, manifesting mainly as hives or itching. Less commonly, patients may experience tightness in the chest and difficulty breathing; very rarely a lifethreatening allergic reaction may occur. IVIg also increases the viscosity of blood, making it more likely to form blood clots. This can lead to venous thrombosis and pulmonary embolism, a condition wherein the clots that form in the veins of the legs and pelvis break free and travel to the lungs. Blood clots can also cause heart attacks and strokes. Even if there are no overt blood clots, the increased blood viscosity can cause kidney failure. Fortunately, these serious complications are rare, but they do need to be considered, particularly in diabetics and in older patients, who may have other risk factors for stroke or heart attack, such as high blood pressure, smoking, or high cholesterol.

The studies showing the effectiveness of PLEX and IVIg have raised a therapeutic dilemma. Ideally, treatment should be started within 2 weeks of onset in order to have maximum the likelihood of an effective outcome. However, some patients are only mildly affected by GBS and may not need treatment. Attempts to identify patients who are likely to develop severe weakness, and therefore need IVIg or PLEX, have so far been only partially successful. It is probably unnecessary to treat mildly affected individuals who are still able to walk without support and those with restricted forms of the disease, such as the Miller Fisher syndrome, but it is important to follow all of them closely to monitor progression. If progression is rapid, treatment could be started earlier. In addition, when the antecedent event is of a type known to be associated with severe disease or when there is a short duration between the antecedent event and the onset of neurologic symptoms, which also may anticipate severe disease, the threshold for beginning treatment may be lower. As with any therapeutic decision, the possible risks of treatment must be weighed against the risks of the disease itself.

IVIg is safe and effective in the treatment of severe GBS, and is easier to use and has fewer side effects than PLEX. It can be used in all age groups, but should be used with caution in the elderly or patients with risk factors for blood clots.

STEROID TREATMENT

Corticosteroid medications, such as cortisone and prednisone, were first used to treat GBS in the early 1950s. Initial reports indicated that they were effective. However, the chronic form of demyelinating neuropathy, CIDP, was not distinguished from GBS during that era. In retrospect, many of the patients who responded to the treatment probably had CIDP. Small controlled studies done during the 1970s showed no beneficial effect; in fact, the patients who received prednisone did slightly worse than the patients who received no treatment. Further studies were done as recently as the late 1990s, using different formulations of steroids and different routes of administration, and again no benefit was shown. One would think that all the evidence against the beneficial effects of steroids would have eliminated their use. However, some patients are still receiving prednisone or some other steroid for the treatment for GBS. The authors strongly recommend that GBS patients *not* receive any form of steroid treatment for their GBS. These medications are ineffective and have many risks, some of which are severe and even life threatening.

Steroid medications should not be used in the treatment of GBS.

FUTURE THERAPEUTIC DIRECTIONS

Despite our best efforts, about 5 percent of GBS patients die from the disease or its complications, and another 10 to 20 percent make an incomplete recovery. Furthermore, the current therapeutic options are far from ideal. They are extremely expensive, inconvenient to administer, and carry some risk. New therapies are, therefore, much needed.

In an attempt to enhance recovery, GBS patients have been treated with a trophic factor called *brain-derived neurotrophic factor* (BDNF). Trophic factors are known to support and enhance nerve regeneration in experimental animals. Unfortunately, BDNF has not improved the outcome in patients with GBS. Thus, there are no new treatments on the horizon for the unfortunate minority of GBS patients who have an incomplete recovery. Better efforts need to be made to recognize the disease in its earliest stages, so that appropriate treatment can be instituted in a timely fashion. Early treatment appears to improve outcome.

CHAPTER 8

Life After Guillain-Barré Syndrome

As mentioned throughout this book, most Guillain-Barré syndrome A(GBS) patients have a good outcome. They recover, resume their previous activities, and put their experience with GBS behind them. However, both during recovery and thereafter, several issues may come up. This chapter addresses several of these matters as well as some of the unique issues facing children with GBS and their parents. In addition, patients who do not completely recover may have other challenges to face, which are also addressed in this chapter.

PAIN

Pain is an underappreciated symptom that may persist for many years after GBS. It may be neuropathic pain or the pain that results from overuse of incompletely recovered muscles. Pain also occurs during the paralytic phase of the illness, as has been discussed previously (see Chapter 2).

Neuropathic Pain

Pain is an important defense mechanism that prevents us from injuring ourselves. If you put your hand in a flame, receptors in the skin perceive the heat and rapidly transmit that information to the brain so that the hand is withdrawn before serious injury can occur. This physiologic pain is called *nociceptive pain.* However, the nerve fibers that transmit these messages in a normal situation may be damaged in any neuropathic disease, including GBS, resulting in neuropathic pain. This type of pain does not have any protective function. The message that the damaged nerve fibers send to the brain is really an illusion, although the pain is certainly real. Neuropathic pain usually emerges as the other manifestations of the acute attack of GBS are subsiding. Pain that occurs during the acute stage of the illness is usually nociceptive, arising from the pain receptors in the lining of the nerve bundles, probably activated by inflammation.

Severe, disabling neuropathic pain is rare, but many patients complain of persistent discomfort in their feet. This discomfort may take the form of tingling, an illusion of swelling or tightness, or a vague, aching pain. Occasionally, there is more severe burning or stabbing pain. It may be associated with marked sensitivity to touch, so that even the light touch of the bed sheets is perceived as painful. The symptoms tend to be worse in the evening or at night and may disturb sleep, exacerbating fatigue. Neuropathic pain is particularly annoying during the nights that follow days during which the patients have been on their feet, and the resulting lack of sleep may interfere with rehabilitation. Pain improves with time in some patients, but others are left with annoying or even disabling pain that persists for years, sometimes for the remainder of the patient's life.

Even though most patients recover their strength following GBS, some are left with persistent pain. This is usually only an annoyance, but occasionally it can be severe. It tends to subside with time but can be permanent.

Treatment of Neuropathic Pain

Treatment of neuropathic pain is a major challenge. Complete relief is difficult to achieve; usually the best that can be hoped for is to make the pain tolerable. It is important that the patient understand this because expectations are important in defining satisfaction with treatment. The patient will be disappointed if they expect complete pain relief and achieve only a 50 percent reduction, although the treating physician may feel satisfied that this is the best result possible. The patient who expects only some improvement will be more satisfied with a mere 50 percent reduction. Since the pain is usually worse at night and sleep disturbance is one of its most disabling aspects, the primary goal should be to improve sleep. Neuropathic pain always seems worse when one is lying awake in the dark of night. Patients repeatedly say such things as: "I can tolerate the pain during the day if I can sleep through the night." Neuropathic pain often leads to depression, and the second goal of treatment is to manage any mood disorder. Pain always feels worse when a person is depressed. Thus, sleep disturbance and depression need to be treated in conjunction with the pain itself. The overall goal is to improve quality of life.

Neuropathic pain does not respond well to simple analgesics such as acetaminophen (Tylenol®) and aspirin, or even to narcotics such as morphine, although narcotics may be needed in some instances. While single drugs are frequently tried, combinations of different drugs are often needed. Table 8-1 shows a partial list of the drugs commonly used to treat neuropathic pain in GBS. Often, it is a matter of "trial and error" to find the drug or combination of drugs that works best for an individual. All of these medications, except the simple analgesics, have to be taken on a daily basis to be effective. One factor in deciding whether to treat residual pain is that it is usually rather mild. Thus, patients may be irritated daily by their symptoms, but be reluctant to take a drug every day for a symptom that significantly bothers them only once or twice a week. Furthermore, these drugs are only partially effective and may need to be given at high doses. A common side effect of all of the medications used in the treatment of neuropathic pain is tiredness. This can be disabling in patients who are already likely to be suffering some degree of fatigue.

Many physicians start with a tricyclic antidepressant (TCA) drug such as nortriptyline for the treatment of neuropathic pain. Older patients and diabetics are more likely to experience side effects with TCA drugs and they may not be the best choice in these patients. The common side effects of TCA drugs, listed in Table 8-2, are dry mouth, sedation, confusion (particularly in the elderly), constipation, difficulty initiating urination (particularly in an older man who may have an enlarged prostate), erectile dysfunction, and dizziness when standing too quickly because the blood pressure falls too low. Less commonly, irregular heartbeat may occur. The dose should be started low (10 to 25 mg) and given in the evening shortly before bedtime. Given at this time, the sedating effects can be beneficial in helping sleep. The dose can then be slowly increased until intolerable side effects occur or a satisfactory relief of symptoms is achieved. Typical effective doses are 75 to 125 mg daily, but many people cannot tolerate doses this high. Nortriptyline is also an antidepressant medication, so it has three potential benefits: pain relief, sleep enhancement, and relief of depression. If nortriptyline is ineffective or cannot be tolerated, it is probably not worth trying other TCA drugs because they will have the same drawbacks and are no more effective.

Table 8-1. Drugs Used in the Treatment of Neuropathic Pain

1. Tricyclic antidepressant drugs:
- Amitriptyline (Elavil®)
- Nortriptyline (Pamelor®)
- Imipramine

2. Other antidepressant drugs:
- Duloxetine (Cymbalta®)
- Venlafaxine (Effexor®)
- Bupropion (Wellbutrin®)

3. Antiepileptic drugs:
- Gabapentin (Neurontin®)
- Carbamazepine (Tegretol®)
- Oxcarbazepine (Trileptal®)
- Tiagabine (Gabitril®)
- Pregabalin (Lyrica®)

4. Narcotic drugs:
- Fentanyl (Duragesic patches)
- Oxycodone controlled release (Oxycontin®)
- Morphine controlled release (MS Contin®)
- Methadone

Paradoxically, the TCA drugs that have been available for several decades seem to more effective than the newer antidepressants for treating neuropathic pain. The newer medications are preferred for the treatment of depression because they are more effective and have fewer side effects. However, pain can increase when a well-meaning primary care physician changes the medication from nortriptyline to sertraline (Zoloft®) or fluoxetine (Prozac®) in an attempt to reduce the side effects of the tricyclic medications. Some recent studies suggest that the newer drugs, such as venlafaxine (Effexor®) and bupropion (Wellbutrin®), may well have some benefit for neuropathic pain independent of their antidepressant effects. The newest of these antidepressant drugs, duloxetine (Cymbalta®), has been approved by the Food and Drug Administration (FDA) for diabetic neuropathic pain and for depression. If a patient is suffering from neuropathic pain and significant depression, and the depression is not satisfactorily controlled with nortriptyline, the addition of another antidepressant is indicated. It seems sensible to use duloxetine because it may have the dual effect of reducing pain and improving mood.

Table 8-2. Side Effects of Drugs Used in the Treatment of Neuropathic Pain

1. Tricyclic antidepressant drugs:
- Sedation
- Confusion
- Dizziness
- Dry mouth
- Constipation
- Urinary retention
- Impotence
- Irregular heart beat
- Low blood pressure

2. Other antidepressant drugs:
- Sedation
- Reduced libido (sex drive)

3. Antiepileptic drugs:
- Sedation
- Dizziness
- Indigestion/heartburn
- Swollen ankles

4. Narcotic drugs:
- Sedation
- Confusion
- Constipation
- Addiction/habituation

Another choice for treating neuropathic pain is an antiepileptic drug such as gabapentin (Neurontin®). For many physicians this is the first choice for the elderly or for patients who otherwise are deemed likely to be unable to tolerate nortriptyline. Gabapentin is added slowly to the nortriptyline, which is usually continued at a lower dose. The most common side effects are sedation and dizziness; sedation is more common but usually abates with time despite continuing the same dose. Dizziness is more disabling and is the most common reason people stop taking gabapentin. Once again, the dose should be started low (300 mg at bedtime in patients under 60 years of age and 100 mg in those 60 or older) and increased slowly until the desired effect is achieved or intolerable adverse effects occur. Most patients notice some improvement at 300 mg three times daily, but the benefit is usually not sustained at this dose. The dose can be increased up to as much as 3,600 mg a day, divided into three to four doses, if needed. Higher doses are rarely indicated because the body is unable to absorb any more of the drug from the intestine. Unlike nortriptyline, which can be administered in a single dose at bedtime, gabapentin needs to be given three to four times daily. Nortriptyline and gabapentin can be used in combination, although the combined sedative effects may limit dosing. A new anticonvulsant drug called pregabalin (Lyrica®) has recently been approved by the FDA for management of diabetic neuropathic pain. Clinical studies indicate that this drug has considerable promise.

The effectiveness of the drugs that have been tried in the treatment of neuropathic pain can vary greatly. The key is to work with a physician who is willing to try different drugs and drug combinations. It should be emphasized that none of these drugs is approved by the FDA for the treatment of neuropathic pain following GBS. Pregabalin and duloxetine have been FDA approved for pain related to diabetic neuropathy. There is no reason to expect that a drug that is effective for neuropathic pain of one type, such as diabetic neuropathy, would not work for other types of neuropathic pain.

If narcotics are necessary for the treatment of neuropathic pain, long-acting forms should be used. This can be achieved by prescribing a drug such as methadone that has a long duration of action, or by giving sustained-release oral formulations, such as MS Contin® (a form of morphine) or Oxycontin® (a form of oxycodone), or transdermal patches that slowly release the drug from a patch attached to the skin, such as fentanyl (Duragesic®) patches. Short-acting forms of these drugs can be used as a supplement to the long-acting forms. Oxycodone is available in a "lollipop" form that can be used as needed when pain is severe. Concern about addiction to these powerful narcotics is greatly exaggerated, at least for patients with neuropathic pain. Patients are carefully monitored for signs of increased demand for the medication, particularly increasing use of the short-acting forms, because the risk of addiction is higher with the short-acting narcotics. The total dose taken in an average week, rather than the dose on a specific day, is the most important. Neuropathic pain typically fluctuates; some days are worse than others. Physicians should not be concerned if a patient exceeds the prescribed dose once in a while as long as the total cumulative dose over the course of a week, or more, is not consistently increasing. Stopping the narcotics is seldom a problem in cases where severe neuropathic pain has subsided. As with the antidepressant and antiepileptic drugs mentioned above, the long-acting narcotics are usually used on a regular schedule, once or twice a day, rather than just when the pain is severe. The shortacting forms are used for short-term relief.

The most common cause of failure of the drugs used in the management of neuropathic pain is that the dose used is not high enough and the drug is not used for long enough. Most patients will experience side effects if drugs are used in sufficient doses to relieve pain, but the benefit should outweigh the side effects. Another problem is patient expectations; treatment is expected to reduce the pain, but will seldom abolish it. If a patient is expecting to be pain free and there is only a 50 percent reduction in pain intensity, this will be regarded as a treatment failure, and yet it may be about the best that can be expected. Complementary treatments may also help manage pain. It is often useful to visit a pain clinic that takes a holistic approach to the management of pain, utilizing both medication and nonpharmacologic strategies. Conventional medicine has been relatively unsuccessful in treating neuropathic pain, causing many patients to try complementary or at least nonpharmacologic approaches. Acupuncture is very popular, but controlled studies show it to be of little, if any, benefit. Hypnosis and meditation can also be useful. Transcutaneous nerve stimulators are small battery-powered units that deliver rapid, low-intensity electrical impulses. These units seem to benefit some patients. Pain clinics usually combine pharmacologic therapy with a variety of other approaches in order to achieve an improvement in the quality of life for patients experiencing pain.

Neuropathic pain usually subsides with time, but may persist for months or years; occasionally, some pain may persist permanently. When treating neuropathic pain, it is important to periodically attempt a reduction in medication to see if it is still needed. While drug combinations are often necessary, simply adding new drugs to the mix without attempting to stop the older ones can lead to increasing adverse effects. An attempt to reduce or stop nortriptyline should be made if a patient on nortriptyline achieves excellent pain relief when gabapentin is added. This may not be successful, but it is worth trying to avoid the inevitable adverse effects of high doses of multiple drugs. Similarly, if a patient has been on a drug combination for months or even years, and their pain is minor, an attempt should be made to reduce or stop medication to see if it is still necessary.

Many medications can reduce neuropathic pain, but high doses and drug combinations are often needed, which can lead to inevitable side effects. The goal is to improve quality of life rather than to simply abolish pain.

Pain From Overuse

Pain can occur in tendons, ligaments, and around joints as a result of overuse in those patients who have residual weakness. Strong muscles are critical in maintaining the stability of joints; when the muscles are weak, the joints become lax, putting strain on the surrounding structures, leading to chronic pain. Unlike neuropathic pain, overuse pain is made worse by activity, particularly walking. It is relieved by rest and seldom disturbs sleep. It is usually an aching felt deep within the limb rather than a burning or shooting pain. Overuse pain is common as a temporary manifestation during rehabilitation, but tends to subside as the muscles strengthen. It may persist if weakness remains.

The most common residual weakness is around the ankles, leading to foot drop and a tendency to turn and twist the ankles; this is the most common site of overuse pain. Less commonly, it may affect the small joints of the hands. The disturbance of gait that can result from residual foot drop can also lead to chronic hip and low back pain. Judicious use of foot braces will help stabilize the ankles and limit these symptoms. The most common form of brace is a plastic brace molded to the foot that fits inside the shoe (molded ankle-foot orthosis [MAFO]; *see* Figure 6-1). Some people prefer the MAFO to be hinged at the ankle so there can be movement in a back and forth plane with good lateral stability.

Unlike neuropathic pain, overuse pain does not respond to antiepileptic or antidepressant drugs, but does respond to anti-inflammatory drugs such as naproxen and ibuprofen. These drugs can cause indigestion or heartburn and occasionally stomach ulcers. Medication to counteract gastric side effects can be prescribed if indigestion or heartburn is a problem with anti-inflammatory drugs.

FATIGUE

Persistent residual fatigue following the acute paralytic illness is one of the most common complaints of GBS patients, and yet it has garnered very little research effort; most of the early studies on the ultimate outcome of GBS do not even mention it. Many of these studies are based on telephone interviews or chart reviews done long after the patient has been discharged from the care of the neurologist, and seemingly minor complaints may have been missed or disregarded. For example, patients may be asked if they have returned to their former work or other previous activities, but they may not have been specifically asked whether they have more difficulty performing those activities. An individual may be back at work, but may be struggling to do their job because of fatigue.

The first note of caution regarding the completeness of recovery was sounded in a small study by Dr. J. McLeod and his colleagues in Australia. These researchers objectively evaluated a small group of 18 recovered GBS patients, and found that half of them had abnormalities on neurologic examination, not 15 to 25 percent as previous publications suggested. The residual objective findings were seemingly trivial, but may still have resulted in greater than normal difficulty in performing the tasks of every day living. A few years later, in 1990, Drs. D.S. Burrows and A.C. Cuetter reported on four patients with persistent lack of stamina, even after muscle strength and electrophysiologic (EMG) studies had returned to normal. All of these patients were Armed Forces personnel who had been assessed annually prior to their GBS using the Army Physical Fitness Test (APFT), a measure of neuromuscular endurance rather than raw muscle strength, as assessed during the standard neurologic examination. Each patient had suffered from GBS of moderate severity, and each was judged to have made a full recovery in terms of muscle strength. However, their APFT had not returned to their former level 1 to 4 years after the acute illness.

A more recent report from Dr. I.S.J. Merkies and his colleagues in Holland has established that the residual effects of GBS are much more common than has been generally reported, and that seemingly minor neurologic symptoms may still be disabling. This study used an index of fatigue severity to assess residual disability. It included 83 patients who had suffered from GBS an average of 5 years previously. About 80 percent of these patients reported fatigue that was considered severe enough to interfere with their life despite the fact that the majority had normal strength or only minor weakness. They noted that the fatigue did not seem to improve over time; it was the same for patients in whom many years had elapsed since their acute attack as it was in patients whose acute illness had occurred only 6 to 12 months previously. They also found that there was little correlation between the degree of residual weakness and the degree of fatigue. These reports support the validity of the observations of many patients who complain of fatigue even when they have returned to all or most of their former activities, including working full time at their former jobs. Although their strength may be normal when they are examined in the doctor's office, they are clearly unable to sustain the same level of physical activity they had performed prior to GBS. Confirmation of these results is needed.

It is important to manage fatigue through energy conservation strategies. GBS patients need to learn how to pace themselves in all that they do. They must schedule time for physical and mental rest during their daily activities. Cooperative, understanding family members and employers can make this strategy easier. It is equally important to consult with a neurologist, physiatrist, or other physician who truly understands the issues that arise following GBS. This individual can advocate for the patient in getting accommodations at work, and explain to family members that the patient really is still affected by GBS even though they may look normal.

Paradoxically, exercise is a key component of any energy conservation strategy. Recent studies have shown that a careful exercise program can reduce fatigue in GBS and chronic inflammatory demyelinating polyneuropathy (CIDP) patients. This may seem counterproductive for someone who is already feeling tired; however, avoidance of exercise leads to deconditioning and an increase in fatigue. "Little and often" should be the GBS patient's focus when exercising, not "no pain, no gain." During any exercise period, the patient should take a break every few minutes to replace fluids and sit down for a few minutes before resuming exercise. Initially, an exercise program may consist of as little as 5 minutes of exercise and 5 minutes of rest, repeated 2 to 3 times. Exercise can be increased as stamina improves, but frequent rest periods are still needed. Exercise should be done at least 3 days a week, but probably not every day. Consultation with a rehabilitation physician or physical therapist to discuss energy conservation strategies may be very useful. It is also important to consider the possible role of depression in causing, or at least exacerbating, fatigue because depression can be treated.

There are no medications proven to be effective in treating fatigue in GBS patients. There are a number of agents that have been studied in multiple sclerosis (MS), another autoimmune demyelinating disease in which fatigue is a major problem. Amantadine, a drug initially introduced as an antiviral agent to treat influenza (it did not work) has been shown to improve fatigue in MS patients, but a recent study showed that it was ineffective in GBS patients with residual fatigue. Stimulants such as modafinil (Pro-vigil®), methylphenidate (Ritalin®), or even dextroamphetamine (Dexedrine®) are also used in MS with some benefit, and may warrant use in some GBS cases. None of these agents has been studied in GBS, and if they are tried, they need to be used with caution.

Fatigue is a common residual symptom in GBS even if strength has been fully recovered. The impact of fatigue can be minimized by energy conservation strategies and judicious exercise.

EMOTIONAL PROBLEMS AFTER ACUTE GBS

The emotional impact of acute GBS on patients and their families is covered in Chapter 2. However, this emotional impact may persist long after the patient has been discharged from neurologic care. Patients dealing with residual effects of the acute disease, such as weakness, pain, and fatigue, may also battle depression. Anxiety about a possible recurrence is also common despite constant reassurance that the disease almost never returns. These worries are experienced by the patient and the entire family. Financial hardships may have resulted from the illness and may persist for many years, especially if the patient has been unable to return to work. Depression is particularly common if the patient has been unable to return to work or other former activities. These symptoms are more severe in patients with incomplete recovery, but are also experienced by those who have apparently recovered fully. There may be obvious symptoms of anxiety and depression, but the effects may be more subtle and yet lead to disturbed sleep, loss of appetite or excessive eating, loss of sex drive *(libido)* and avoidance of intimacy, and a general loss of interest in activities that were formerly enjoyed. All family members need to be aware of the symptoms of anxiety and depression, and medical consultation should be sought if necessary. Treatment with medication or with individual or family psychotherapy can be extremely helpful. Most antidepressant medications are also effective for anxiety; the newer drugs have a very low incidence of serious adverse effects.

LONG-TERM EXPECTATIONS FOR RECOVERY

Prognosis for Adults

As stated previously, the overall outlook for the GBS patient is relatively optimistic. Although the exact percentages vary from study to study, the following values give an estimate for long-term prognosis:

1. Approximately 75 percent of patients have full recovery of strength. Some of them may have persisting but mild abnormalities that will not interfere with long-term function. These may include abnormal sensations such as tingling, mild pain, or loss of stamina.
2. Fifteen to 20 percent of patients have long-term modest disabilities; examples include unsteady walking, and the need to compensate for this with the use a cane, or persistent footdrop warranting the use of an MAFO to improve walking (see Figure 6-1). These patients may be able to return to most or all of their former activities, depending on their former work and life style.
3. Five to 10 percent of patients will have severe, long-term disability that will prevent a return to their prior life style or occupation. Some, for ex-

ample, may require the long-term use of a wheelchair, walker, or crutches.

Time to Recovery

The time it takes to recover depends primarily on the severity of the paralysis. In some patients, progression stops after a week or less; they never lose the ability to walk and will have returned to normal within a month or two. Patients may become completely paralyzed in more severe cases, and may not even begin to improve until 2 to 3 months after the onset of weakness. Once recovery begins, it typically proceeds rapidly at first, as demyelinated axons reconstitute their myelin sheath. The pace of recovery then slows as damaged axons regenerate, a much slower and less efficient process. Most recovery occurs within about 2 to 3 years from the onset of GBS. The literature implies that minimal, if any, recovery occurs after 2 to 3 years; however, many patients relate continued recovery well after that, although the additional improvements may be minor. Nevertheless, there may be a role for ongoing regular exercise to help strengthen weaker muscles. Certainly, functioning can improve even if strength does not.

The rate and degree of recovery can be predicted to some extent. As one would expect, patients with the most severe paralysis make the slowest and poorest recovery. Data from the North American GBS Study Group indicate that patients with the following findings have an excellent (95 percent) chance of recovery, defined as being able to walk unassisted within 3 months of the beginning of their illness:

- Relatively preserved muscle responses to electrical stimulation of the motor nerves
- Received plasmapheresis within 4 weeks of beginning of symptoms
- Did not need a respirator to support breathing
- Did not see a doctor until after 7 days of symptoms (implying that their illness developed more slowly)
- Young age (closer to 30 than 60 years of age)

The following characteristics predicted poor recovery: only a 10 percent chance at 3 months and a 20 percent chance at 6 months of walking unassisted:

- Low amplitude (size) of the muscle responses to electrical stimulation of motor nerves
- Did not receive plasmapheresis within 4 weeks of onset of symptoms
- Needed a ventilator to support breathing
- Saw a doctor within 7 days of onset of symptoms (implying that their illness came on rapidly)
- Older age (closer to 60 than 30 years of age)

Prognosis for Children

Little has been written about children with GBS, and even less about the special challenges involved. Most studies indicate that the outcome for children with GBS is excellent. A Dutch study reported in the late 1990s indicated that patterns of recovery in children are similar to that of young adults in their 30s, as described above. Guidelines for the family of a child with GBS are outlined in Chapter 2, and will not be discussed here except to emphasize that the recovering child with GBS or the child with active CIDP can have an impact on the entire family. Some aspects specific to living with the residual effects of GBS in a child include the following.

Fatigue and the Child's World

As with adults, fatigue may be an enduring symptom in children, at least during the first few months following the acute paralysis. The child may look normal, and this may create resentment, particularly in siblings. The fatigue will usually improve with time, and family members, friends, teachers, and even medical professionals need to be positive and optimistic. They may need to be educated regarding the frequent and often disabling fatigue of GBS because the uneducated may think the child is pretending to be sick when they say they need to rest. Many of the comments of other family members, friends, and teachers may be well meant, but they can be extremely frustrating, both for the child and the parents. Be polite, firm, and matter-of-fact with the people in your child's world about the child's need to rest: "Yes, she really is that tired." "Yes, she could walk this morning, but this afternoon she needs to use the wheelchair." "Yes, we really need to use handicapped parking." "No, herbs and yoga cannot replace physical therapy." "No, she is not crazy and we are not in denial."

Situations may come up during recovery that will challenge the judgment of the parent and physician. For example, the child may show more energy, but will she have enough endurance to continue home schooling and also rejoin the Girl Scouts or the church choir? As concerned parents we do not want our children to miss out on the experiences of childhood. But children often try to push the limits even if they are not strong enough. This is only natural. Parents need to monitor their child's tolerance for activity so they do not overextend themselves prematurely.

Children Are Capable of Participating in Care Decisions

Children are more likely to respond positively to choices and make more realistic ones if they are allowed to participate in the decision-making process. Try to avoid being condescending; the child knows his or her own body better than anyone else, and may be in the best position to know what he or she can endure. Taking the child out of the loop of decision making can only add to their resentment and frustration with being sick. Little issues may still be important. Questions to ask the child may include: "Which shoes feel most comfortable? Before you return to school next week, should you ask your teacher to explain to your class why you might get tired and need to rest? Should we make plans for next week's field trip in case you become exhausted? Should we explain to your friends that the scar in the front of your neck is from the tracheostomy? Would you like to wear turtle necks until you feel more comfortable about explaining the scar?"

Undergoing frequent plasma exchange or intravenous gamma globulin treatments, which involve needle sticks, can become a real problem, especially for the CIDP patient. This is also an issue for the hospitalized child with GBS. Pain is usually felt as the needle penetrates the skin, and there may be additional pain if the needle has to be manipulated to get it into a vein. Stress may be reduced if the patient is allowed to provide input. For example, the skill involved in the insertion of a needle varies among medical caregivers. Some are gentle; some are rough. An injection of local anesthetic under the skin will numb the skin, but it often burns upon initial injection; this can last half a minute. Pain from this procedure can be reduced by neutralizing the acidic local anesthetic with about 10 percent volume of sodium bicarbonate, which is available commercially in a strength of 34 percent. Use the smallest needle that will do the job effectively; a 30-gauge needle will produce less pain than a larger gauge needle. Local anesthetic can also be applied to the skin to reduce pain, but it does not penetrate very far, and it may need to be combined with the injection to get adequate pain relief. The patient, having had prior experiences, may be able to offer the technician, nurse, or doctor details about needle sticks, including where the best veins are located; when the local anesthetic has numbed the skin so a needle can be inserted without causing pain; or whether they have a tendency to faint from a needle stick and that lying down first is warranted. The patients' involvement in their care will give them some feeling of control and reduce their anger or resentment about their situation.

Education

It is likely that schooling will be interrupted for the child with GBS or CIDP. When the child is diagnosed with GBS, usually in the hospital, the duration of their illness may perhaps be estimated, but not with certainty. They may be able to return to school in the fall if the illness began in June at the end of the school year; however, residual fatigue is likely to affect their education. Parents should inform the school system of the child's illness, and plan for alternatives to in-school education. A note from the doctor giving the diagnosis and, if possible, an estimate of how long the illness will last may be helpful to the child's educators. Remember that the weakness of GBS improves in a descending pattern, so the child may be able to write before they can walk. A child can go to class, even in a wheelchair, if transportation is available. Of course, the emotional impact of such a scenario should be considered before proceeding with this option.

Obligations of the School System. Public Law 94-142 mandates a "free and appropriate education for every child in the least restrictive environment." Many, but not all, school systems have options to educate a home-bound child or one with disabilities. Budgetary considerations may limit the services that a particular community or school system is willing or able to offer. It is best to be your child's advocate in such situations. Learn what their physical and educational needs are and pursue the best possible schooling.

An Individual Educational Plan can be created for your child. This type of plan can be changed as your child improves and discontinued when there is enough recovery to return to normal schooling. Even if your local school system does not offer the services your child needs, they may be mandated under law to utilize such services from a neighboring community's school system. Again, if resistance is met, be firm but polite in reinforcing their obligations to comply with the law.

Planning the School Day. Public schools are required to provide accommodations for a child's disabilities as long as it is feasible without risking the child's health. Usually, once a child is home from rehabilitation, they will be able to return to their education. This may be at home or at their regular school, depending upon their particular situation. Schools are expected to make accommodations so students can participate in activities such as field trips, marching bands, and stage performances even if they use a wheelchair or crutches. Physical education classes can be modified to meet a child's needs. For example, physical education class can be replaced with a rest period so the child will be attentive for the rest of the day's academic classes. Perhaps a formal rehabilitation exercise program set up by the child's therapists can be implemented later in the day.

Accommodations for Remaining Weakness. By the time a child is ready to go back to school, their hands may still be too weak to write and a computer can be a practical alternative. Tests can be given orally or the answers spoken into a recorder. Tests requiring an answer to be circled or checked may be easier than a written reply. However, if the child lacks dexterity, the places to put check marks or circles should be far enough apart so the student's answer is clearly indicated. If the child is able to walk but requires crutches or a cane, someone can volunteer or be designated on a rotating basis to carry the child's books and lunch tray. If fatigue is a major problem, a prolonged lunch period may be a solution so the patient can nap in a quiet place after eating, such as the infirmary or lounge.

ABNORMAL SENSATIONS

As they recover from the paralysis of Guillain-Barré syndrome and become more active, some patients notice that continuous activity, such as walking, will bring on abnormal sensations, including tingling of the toes or fingers, and further activity will lead to fatigue and even collapse. These abnormal sensations act as an early marker of impending fatigue. The patient should use this type of warning as a signal to sit down and rest. The fatigue and tingling usually fade with time.

RECURRENCE OF SYMPTOMS SIMILAR TO GBS

Some patients develop a mild recurrence of their GBS symptoms months or even years after their initial illness. Not surprisingly, this leads to great concern that the GBS is recurring. Although GBS can recur, it is extremely rare, and these recurrent symptoms are almost always benign. Recurrent weakness or tingling should not be equated with recurrent GBS. There are a number of possible explanations for this phenomenon. Most commonly it is due to incomplete recovery of damaged nerves. The myelin sheath does not always return completely to normal when the nerve recovers. It may function normally in most circumstances, but under stress it may decompensate, leading to the return of the initial symptoms. Many different stresses can cause this decompensation, including raised body temperature from a fever caused by infection, exercising in a warm environment, or taking a long, hot bath. Other possible stresses include dehydration, concurrent medical illness, such as a cold or the flu, and any change in medications. Many patients note that just getting exhausted from trying to do too much or even emotional stress can make their initial symptoms reappear. Only strong reassurances will be needed if the recurrence of symptoms is transient.

Seek medical advice if the recurrent symptoms last for more than 24 hours because other causes will need to be considered. Many of the symptoms of GBS are nonspecific, and can also occur with a large number of other neurologic and medical disorders. For example, the patient may have developed another neurologic illness, such as carpal tunnel syndrome, or they may have developed a medical illness, such as thyroid deficiency, vitamin deficiency, or diabetes, that has caused the recurrent symptoms. The initial diagnosis may have been wrong, and the patient may really have chronic inflammatory demyelinating polyneuropathy (CIDP), a related but chronic disorder that is discussed in Chapter 9. CIDP may be indistinguishable from GBS at the time of initial presentation. It responds to the same treatment as GBS, only to relapse when the treatment is stopped, or sometimes months or even years later. Another electrophysiologic study may be needed, and possibly a repeat lumbar puncture if CIDP is suspected. The least likely explanation for recurrent symptoms is a second attack of GBS. Although exceedingly rare, this does happen.

One mechanism of recurrent weakness following GBS may be analogous to the post-polio syndrome. Poliomyelitis typically occurs in childhood or early adulthood. Individuals who have had polio may recover completely, but often there is some residual permanent weakness. It has long been recognized that patients who have mild, stable weakness following their initial attack of polio can deteriorate decades later. This condition is called *post-polio syndrome.* It is not due to the return of the polio virus, and its mechanism is controversial. The most plausible explanation is that there is age-related attrition of an already depleted pool of motor nerves. Some motor nerve cells are destroyed by the virus during an acute episode of polio. Recovery of strength occurs because the surviving motor nerves take over the muscle fibers originally supplied by the destroyed nerves. In this way, some function is restored, but there will be fewer motor nerve cells. All of us lose nerve cells with the passage of time, but most of us have a surplus so that we do not become weak. When an individual has had polio, the normal process of nerve cell loss leads to increased weakness in previously stable muscles because a surplus does not exist. It has been suggested that a similar phenomenon occurs in patients who have had GBS. In the early 1990s, the GBS Foundation took an informal poll of patients who thought they had developed a post-GBS syndrome. About 30 responses were obtained. Of these, almost all of them were found to have some other explanation for their complaints—based on the information provided. Most were found to be experiencing the persistence of weakness, fatigue, and/or sensation problems that they had initially experienced as part of their GBS. In summary, the informal poll did not identify a recurrence of GBS-like symptoms that would fit into the concept of a situation similar to the post-polio syndrome; that is, a "post-GBS syndrome." This is not to say that it does not occur; however, it is imperative to exclude other causes of new weakness in previously stable muscles before attributing it to post-GBS syndrome.

SAFETY OF IMMUNIZATIONS

Flu shots and other immunizations are usually safe for patients who have had GBS. Immunizations rarely cause significant side effects, and the illnesses they are used to prevent often lead to serious complications. GBS can occur following certain vaccinations. As mentioned previously, rabies inoculation has long been known to cause GBS in some individuals. The notorious swine influenza vaccination program has also been established as having caused several hundred cases of GBS. One polio vaccination program possibly caused a few cases of GBS. Other than these examples, it is remarkable how rare it is for vaccination to precipitate GBS. Also, there are probably individuals whose GBS was precipitated by a specific vaccine, as discussed in the section on molecular mimicry in Chapter 4. The question is whether having had GBS makes it likely that the disease will recur if a vaccination is given. The answer is a resounding *NO.* There is no evidence whatsoever indicating that an individual who has had GBS is at any increased risk for developing another attack of

GBS following a vaccination even if the initial event was precipitated by a vaccine. No two vaccines are the same, and the likelihood that an individual would develop an identical illness following two separate vaccinations is small.

The risk of complications from the flu is substantial, and that risk is markedly greater than the very small risk of developing GBS from a flu vaccination. For example, in patients over the age of 65 years, as many as 10,000 persons per million have required hospitalization because of the flu, with a death rate as high as 1,500 per million. In contrast, the average number of GBS cases in the general population is less than 2 per 100,000 each year, with a mortality or death rate of only 3 percent within that small group. Thus, the risk of developing a significant complication from the flu is much greater than the risk of developing GBS. For these reasons, it is generally recommended that patients who fulfill the standard criteria to receive a flu shot should do so. For all vaccinations, the risk must be weighed against the benefit.

Even though there is a relatively high risk of getting GBS following rabies vaccination, if one is bitten by a rabid animal, the chances of dying of rabies if not vaccinated is much higher, so the vaccination should be given.

A more realistic example in the United States is the elderly, life-long smoker with emphysema and heart failure who is entering the flu season. Such an individual is quite likely to develop life-threatening complications from the flu, and vaccination should be recommended regardless of whether GBS had followed a previous flu shot. Conversely, a healthy, young person probably does not need a flu shot, so the benefit is less clear. If that individual had suffered GBS after a previous flu shot, it should probably *not* be repeated. The other issue that needs to be considered to put this controversy into perspective is the risk of developing GBS following the flu. The viral infection itself is probably more likely to cause GBS than the vaccination. If a patient has developed GBS following any vaccination, it is almost impossible to persuade that patient to have any vaccination ever again despite the complete lack of evidence of increased risk. This fear is entirely understandable given the life-threatening and life-altering nature of GBS. Ultimately, each patient who is a candidate for the flu shot or other vaccination should discuss their case with their family physician. Their doctor is in the best position to balance risk against benefit and consider their medical history in order to determine their overall need for the vaccination.

Vaccination for Current and Recent GBS Patients

The guidelines regarding vaccinations are different for patients who are still recovering from GBS. During recovery from GBS, the immune system may be unusually vulnerable to exposure to foreign proteins and viruses. Therefore, some experts recommend against giving an immunization until 6 to 12 months after GBS.

Having had previous GBS does not increase the risk that an individual will have a second attack following subsequent vaccinations even if the first attack occurred following a vaccination. For any individual who has had GBS, it is important to weigh risk and benefit in making a decision about future vaccinations.

INTIMACY

GBS patients going through the process of hospital care and then rehabilitation are usually preoccupied with the process of getting better and have little, if any, interest in physical intimacy. Typically, the physical and emotional demands of this illness take precedence over interest in intimacy. Eventually, as the patient proceeds through the rehabilitation process, interest in intimacy and sexual desire may return. The desire for intimacy varies greatly among individuals, and several factors play a role, including:

- Motivation and interest
- Availability of a partner
- Male *tumescence* (ability to achieve an erection)
- Female arousal

- Sensory integrity of erogenous zones (genitalia and skin, in general)
- Strength and endurance of various muscle groups (pelvis, limbs, and respiratory capacity)
- Gonadal hormonal status
- Nongonadal hormonal status
- Environment/opportunity

Motivation and Interest

Major illness typically has a negative impact on interest in intimacy. Most hospitalized patients are preoccupied with the physical and mental effort of rehabilitation, as well as trying to plan for the future. As patients recover, they usually give more thought to resuming their normal life at home, returning to work, and participating in family and leisure activities. Once home, many GBS patients are still actively undergoing rehabilitation either by attending a day hospital program or being supervised at home by a visiting therapist. Eventually, as the patient's overall strength and endurance improve, a greater interest in intimacy may develop, automatically leading to the resumption of sexual relations.

Some say the brain is the largest sex organ of the body. The point is that the major factor affecting and driving physical desire is the psychological state, attitude, and interest in a partner. These factors are controlled by centers of higher thinking, the brain. Ninety percent of impotency cases in the general population are psychological. A multitude of complex factors underlie the desire for intimacy, a subject far beyond the scope of this book.

Availability of a Partner

Most GBS patients are adults who had a sexual partner prior to getting sick. A smaller group of patients, typically young adults and older teens, may have been actively dating at the time of their illness. Once these patients are well along in recovery—meaning they are able to walk and have substantial endurance—interest in social and intimate relations will likely return.

Physical Ability to Attain and Maintain Tumescence

Impotence is defined as the inability to develop a sufficiently effective erection for intercourse *(coitus).* Fortunately, this is rarely a problem for GBS patients. However, a questionnaire study by Dr. Koppel Burk, a former GBS patient and cardiologist, indicated that some patients experience reduced ability to perform sexual activities after GBS. Published reports indicate that perhaps 1 percent of males who have had GBS will have difficulty attaining and/or maintaining sufficient tumescence to have satisfactory relations. Inadequate tumescence in the GBS patient should be addressed in the same manner as in any other person experiencing impotence. The most common cause of impotence, as already noted, is psychological. Organic causes, such as impaired blood supply to the penis (vasculogenic impotence) or impaired nerve function (neurogenic impotence), account for only about 10 percent of causes of impotence in the general population. In GBS patients, there is a greater chance that impaired nerve function may be a factor. An evaluation for the cause of impotence is commonly done by an urologist, and on occasion by an endocrinologist or the family doctor. A series of questions may readily help determine if impotency is due to an organic or psychological cause, or perhaps a combination. For example, an organic basis for impotency is unlikely if the person develops an erection in the morning on awakening. Medication may be the cause if the impotence began after the start of a new drug.

Organic Causes of Impaired Tumescence

The potential organic causes of impotence include hormonal, vascular (impaired circulation or blood supply), neurologic, and medications. Hormonal causes, which are unlikely in GBS, can be readily checked by measuring blood levels of testosterone and prolactin. Vascular insufficiency or impaired blood supply to the phallus can be readily determined by measuring the penis blood pressure and comparing it to the arm blood pressure. This test can be easily performed by a noninvasive vascular laboratory that is equipped for the study. Poor circulation as a cause of impotence is rarely a problem in GBS.

Penile tumescence requires proper sympathetic nerve function, which can be impaired in GBS. As stated above, the presence of a morning erection prior to voiding is a good marker that the organic components for tumescence are working properly. A penile nocturnal tumescence study is a formal test for nighttime erectile ability. If this study is abnormal, and normal hormone levels and blood supply are found, then neurologic impairment may well be the cause of organic impotence. Some drug types used to treat the complications of GBS have been found to underlie impotence. These include some antihypertensives, stomach acid suppressors (H2 blockers), and anticholinergic-type antidepressants. These drugs can usually be replaced with alternatives without negative side effects.

Male Response: Treatment Options for Impaired Tumescence

Several options are available to treat impotence, including:

- Sildenafil (Viagra®), Vardenafil (Levitra®), and tadalafil (Cialis®) taken by mouth, have been found to be helpful in treating both organic and psychogenic causes.
- A venous flow controller (Actis®) is a device that retains blood in the phallus once tumescence is reached by clamping the base of the phallus.
- A vacuum constriction device.

- Medication that is inserted into the urethra: alprostadil urethral suppository (Muse®).
- Medication that is injected into the penis: alprostadil (Caverject® and Edex®).
- Penile prostheses or implants include those that are semirigid and maintain a stiff insert, and also those that can be inflated via an implanted bulb.

A urologist can detail the pros and cons of these various methods.

Female Response

Normal Female Response. Intimacy in the female is quite strongly driven by psychologic factors, with organic issues playing an infrequent role. Organic components of the female sexual response occur in two stages. The first is sexual arousal leading to genital lubrication. Various stimuli (visual and tactile) contribute to female sexual response. The most common factors interfering with response are psychological, including depression and interpersonal conflicts with the sexual partner. Interference with arousal from neurologic causes is uncommon. A gynecologic assessment may be warranted if this is suspected. Psychologic or psychiatric counseling may be needed if no physical reasons for lack of desire are discovered.

The second stage of the female response *(orgasm)* is typically triggered in part by stimulation of the *clitoris,* leading to automatic pelvic muscle contractions, rocking, and feelings of pleasure. Women also derive great satisfaction from closeness in a cherished relationship with a loving partner.

Potential Problems in GBS. The first stage of the female response, arousal and lubrication, and the second stage, pelvic muscle contractions and pleasure perception, can theoretically be affected in GBS. Actual reports of such problems are difficult to find in the medical literature. Damaged sensory nerves may impair the ability of tactile and other stimuli to trigger arousal and lubrication. Fortunately, the sense of touch is rarely affected in GBS. Saliva or nonprescription lubricants may be helpful if the lubrication response is inadequate. Motor nerve problems can limit pelvic muscle activity. This issue has actually been described anecdotally in GBS patients. An understanding partner and employment of additional creative methods beyond traditional vaginal intercourse may help to circumvent the female's limited pelvic muscle activity. Little else is known about the potential for nerve damage to adversely affect sexuality in GBS patients.

Sensory Integrity (Genitalia and Skin, in General)

The sensory ability to detect touch and temperature, distinguish shapes, and perceive hardness versus softness is usually preserved in GBS. Therefore, skin sensation, which is a major component of intimate activity (caressing, kissing, and foreplay) is usually preserved in GBS.

Strength and Endurance of Various Muscle Groups (Pelvis, Limbs, and Respiratory Capacity)

As previously discussed, strength in GBS usually returns in a descending pattern from the upper to the lower body. The arms usually get stronger before the legs. By the time a patient has sufficient interest in resuming an intimate relationship, it is likely that all of the limbs will have regained sufficient strength to enable satisfactory lovemaking. However, not all GBS patients reach full recovery and strength. Fortunately, this is true in only a small number of patients.

Circumventing Fatigue in Intimacy

Recovering GBS patients typically experience some fatigue during activities such as walking. As recovery progresses, endurance usually improves, allowing the patient to be active for longer periods of time before fatigue sets in. Fatigue is typically experienced as weakness of the muscles being used, such as the legs when walking. The patient typically has to sit down because fatigue will eventually lead to collapse if it is ignored.

Fatigue may become a factor during intimate relations for both men and women. For example, traditional coitus positions usually involve the male's repeated, rapid use of all of his limbs and pelvic muscles. These muscles may not have sufficient innervation to facilitate sustained activity in partially recovered GBS patients. If muscle weakness or fatigue limit traditional sexual activity, but tumescence and emotional drive are present, couples may want to use alternatives to traditional coitus as a means of attaining satisfaction. These potential options include female superior position and oral and manual stimulation if the patient is a male. Use your imagination and be adventurous.

Hormonal Status

This has been addressed previously for males. Gonadal hormone deficiency is rarely a problem in females.

Nongonadal Hormonal Status

In addition to the sex hormones, testosterone and estrogen, other hormones play an indirect role in sexual interest and performance. While GBS patients are not any more likely to have these disorders than the general population, it is important to consider factors unrelated to GBS that might contribute to sexual problems.

Environment and Opportunity

Environment and opportunity play a substantial role in a person's interest in and ability to enjoy intimacy. A quiet environment, such as an empty house or apartment, or a room with a door that can be locked, safe from the risk of intruding children or other adults, is certainly helpful. Of course, good body hygiene is important. The partner may assist with hygiene if the GBS patient does not yet have sufficient use of the hands and limbs to perform good self-hygiene.

Intimacy and the Severely Disabled Patient

One particularly delicate subject in the sexual arena is the profoundly disabled patient with sexual urges but no partner to help them. The Association to Aid the Sexual and Relationships of People with a Disability, London, U.K., is a potential resource in addressing this issue. Your urologist or gynecologist will hopefully be able to direct you to local information.

THE SEVERELY DISABLED PATIENT AT HOME

Most GBS patients can expect to return to work within a year or two. Fortunately, only a small number (perhaps less than 5 to 10 percent) will have long-term major disabilities that prevent their return to work and other former activities. Most of these patients will require ongoing assistance by others for day-to-day activities. Small neurologic improvements may occur after 2 years, bringing additional functioning that will improve the quality of life.

The Wheelchair Experience

It is difficult to accurately predict the pace of improvement or ultimate outcome while the patient is in the acute care setting. Once the GBS patient has been medically stabilized and strength has begun to improve, transfer to a short-term acute rehabilitation facility can be arranged. At that time, assessment of mobility needs will begin. If the patient is improving rapidly, the focus will be on returning to independent walking and early discharge to home. If there is severe weakness and slow improvement, preparation for life with a wheelchair will be necessary. Even if the patient does regain the ability to walk, a wheelchair may be necessary for management of fatigue.

If it becomes apparent during acute rehabilitation that independent home living is not going to be possible immediately, the patient will often be transferred to a long-term rehabilitation hospital where training for living with permanent disability will continue. The goal is always to maximize the degree of independence. Initially, the patient in a wheelchair may not be able to transfer out of the chair independently; they may be unable to dress or feed themselves without help or handle toileting and other basic hygiene needs. They may require full-time care, at least for the foreseeable future.

Options for Outpatient Care

A goal of the rehabilitation staff is to return the patient to their home as soon as possible. If the disability is severe, identification of a long-term caregiver is essential, but this can present major problems. Other family members are usually the first to be called on, but they are not always able to fill the needs of the patient. A spouse may need to work to maintain income for the family. Children may be willing to help out, but they also need to live their own lives. Parents may be too old or have their own illnesses to deal with. A patient may not have other family members to provide the necessary care. These situations will be addressed by the social worker or case manager assigned to the patient at the rehabilitation facility. The case manager can refer the patient and their family to the services, facilities, and funding available in their community. They can arrange for home visits by a nurse and social worker, who will assess the patient's home environment, insurance coverage, and other factors in order to find realistic solutions to any issues. The scenarios that a particular patient may face are myriad, as are the potential solutions, so each one is handled on a case by case basis. The rehabilitation hospital has a vested interest in expediting efficient patient discharge. Accordingly, they will be highly motivated to assist the patient in relocating to a suitable facility or to their home.

Potential Sources of Assistance

If developing a suitable discharge plan remains difficult, one approach is to locate the local governmental office that oversees compliance with the Americans with Disabilities Act (ADA) and ask for guidance. Issues of concern to the wheelchair patient may include safe wheelchair-accessible housing, meals, and medical care. Additional services may include benefits available for veterans, including physical aids and equipment (ramps and electric wheelchair), personal care, education, employment, vocational rehabilitation, wheelchair van or comparable transportation, accessibility to arts, sports and leisure events, sex and personal relationships, and legal services.

Assistance can be sought from local politicians, who typically have a sense of responsibility to their constituency. Assisting the disabled often makes good press, and may motivate a politician to demonstrate his commitment to helping the community by helping you. Religious and social organizations, Rotary Club, Salvation Army, and the YMCA and YWCA are also potential sources of assistance.

Options for Living Space

With very rare exceptions, patients restricted to a wheelchair will need a single-level living space. Elevators can be installed to get a wheelchair upstairs, but they are expensive and cumbersome. Furthermore, at least during the first year or two after GBS, there is the hope of improvement of a sufficient degree to become partly or fully independent of the wheelchair and able to use stairs again. Single-floor living can be accomplished in such housing options as a bungalow or ranch house, apartment that is accessible by elevator, or other comparable arrangement. The GBS patient's living space should be equipped with the following:

- Level access or mild ramping
- Doorways that are wider than the standard 2 feet 3 inches to 2 feet 6 inches
- Walls and doors that are configured to assure access by a wheelchair with leg supports; straight access is easiest
- A bathroom with a bath or shower that can be entered either by rolling in or by easy transfer
- Toilet with seat raised to the same height as the top of the wheelchair cushion
- Firmly attached grab bars at the toilet sides and far shower wall for those who have good arm strength and grip; bars should allow ample room to maneuver.

Powered wheelchairs usually require more space than manual ones. Wheelchairs move poorly over carpet, and the floor covering should be smooth; suggested choices are hardwood, linoleum, or perhaps shortpile carpet. Most patients will end up living with a compromise between optimal housing and other factors, including cost, availability, and location of the spouse's job. Moving to an appropriate dwelling will likely provide the best solution, but this may not be financially realistic.

Options for Care Assistance at Home

The amount of care that a wheelchair patient needs at home varies. Patients with good arm use may be able to fend for themselves for hours at a time when their spouse is at work. A nursing aide or other dependable person can stop in to check on the patient. If the patient's arm and hand use is limited, they can still be left alone for an hour or two, or longer, with precautions such as a portable phone for emergencies. A part-time or even full-time personal care attendant may be necessary for individuals who have no family members who are able to assist them.

Respite Care

Caring for a disabled patient can be exhausting and time consuming. Providing the caregiver with a break from time to time can be invaluable in maintaining a high standard of home care. This may entail admitting the patient to a respite or rehabilitation facility, or having intensive home care provided temporarily.

Activities at Home

The wheelchair patient who returns home will have limited mobility, and possibly problems using their hands and fingers. Methods should be sought to fill the time and gain a sense of accomplishment. The personal computer may fill this need. It can usually be used even by a disabled person. The Internet and e-mail can open up an entire avenue of possibilities for communication, exploring information, and employment. Computers can accept input even from the nontypist. A stick held between the teeth can be used to manipulate the keyboard if the patient cannot use their hands to type. Books provide another source of utilizing time; page-turning devices are available if necessary. Audio books are also available.

Mobility and Transport

The GBS patient who is wheelchair dependent by the end of 1 to 2 years after their illness is likely to need the wheelchair indefinitely. Accordingly, methods to optimize its use should be considered. If the patient can self-propel the chair, a lightweight chair made from a modern alloy is best in order to decrease the weight burden. This type of wheelchair is easy to lift in and out of a regular car, and needs much less space to maneuver around the home and other enclosed areas. Even if the patient cannot self-propel, a lightweight chair will be easier for the caregiver to push and put into a car.

A cushion is an essential component of a wheelchair. The preferable type is one that molds to the patient's bottom, as this will reduce the risk of skin breakdown. Another helpful design is inflatable with an egg crate design, which will reduce focal pressure and prevent skin damage.

Electric scooters for the patient who cannot self-propel should be outfitted with a joystick to allow self-use. Even if the patient does not have sufficient hand strength to manipulate the joystick, controls can be fitted to allow maneuvering using head movements, or even by blowing or sucking on a tube attached to the controls.

Vehicles to accommodate a wheelchair or scooter may be of various designs. Decisions about particulars will vary, depending upon the caregiver's strength, the financial situation, and the patient's needs. Options include rear vehicle carriers and vans with electric lift-side ramps. The options for vehicles and accessories for the disabled can be explored through the Internet.

Public transport for the disabled is extremely variable. Kneeling buses are available in some cities. Even if wheelchairs can be loaded onto buses and trains, the patient must still be safely secured with a seat belt and the wheelchair anchored for protection from falling and injury.

Flying

Most airlines can accommodate the wheelchair patient by allowing the patient to roll up to the gangway entrance to the plane—or through the gangway to the entrance of the plane. The patient is then transferred to a slim, rolling chair that can fit through the plane's narrow aisles. In small airports, where there may be no gangway entrance, the patient will be carried up stairs and into the plane (with some possible loss of dignity). Passengers requiring assistance are the first to be boarded and the last to depart, so plan to check in early.

Ample time must be allowed for connections. Airlines should be informed of your needs when booking a flight. Using the toilet is perhaps the biggest potential problem while flying. Long flights can be broken up into two or more shorter flights to allow extra opportunities to use the toilet. If possible, try to have a bowel movement before boarding the aircraft and avoid the use of laxatives during the 24 hours before the flight. Fluid intake should be restricted before and during flying to reduce the need to urinate. However, the aircraft cabin is a dry environment and flying is dehydrating, so some fluid intake during long flights is necessary. Smaller, frequent drinks will quench thirst and supply the body with steady hydration. Be prepared to make the bathroom the first stop after exiting the airplane. Alcohol is dehydrating and should be avoided immediately before and during a flight.

COMPLEMENTARY THERAPIES

The medical profession has, to some extent, failed patients with residual disabilities from GBS, leading them to seek out alternative therapies. Treatment of the acute illness lies squarely in the realm of conventional medicine: skilled nursing, ventilator support, intravenous immunoglobulin (IVIg), and plasmapheresis. If any residual effects of GBS remain for more than a few months, many patients seek alternative therapies, partly because the conventional medical therapies are not effective. The medical profession usually cannot accelerate the pace of improvement in strength; cannot eliminate numbness or tingling; can only partly relieve pain; and has largely ignored fatigue. Patients do not want to be told that they must wait for healing to happen naturally. They want to get better as quickly as possible. They may be frustrated that the medical profession, which has made so many advances over the last 100 years or so, is unable to restore them to their former life style.

The therapies discussed are of unproven benefit, but fortunately they are not harmful. Research has established that most patients use alternative therapies for their illnesses, but that they usually do so in addition to their medically prescribed therapy. Research has also shown that patients usually do not tell their physician about the alternative therapies they receive. The physician has a responsibility to make every attempt to determine exactly which alternative therapies the patient is using because those therapies may interact with medical treatment. For example, St. John's wort, a widely used herbal remedy that has been shown to have important antidepressant properties, may interact with anticoagulant medication (blood thinners).

Practitioners of alternative medicine, some of whom are physicians, have a lot to teach conventional medical doctors about how to interact with patients because they are often more sympathetic and empathetic. They are more sensitive to the needs of the patient and easier to talk to. Some of the alternative approaches that may be used include the following.

Acupuncture

Originating in China over 2,000 years ago, the popularity of this treatment in America began when a *New York Times* reporter, James Reston, wrote about his doctors in China using it to ease his pain after surgery. A National Institutes of Health (NIH) report indicates that acupuncture has shown benefit in treating postoperative dental pain, low back pain, and carpal tunnel syndrome, and that it may be helpful as an adjunctive therapy to decrease the amount of painkilling drugs required after surgery. Just what role it may have for GBS patients is unclear. It is worth considering for the GBS patient with neuropathic pain that has incompletely responded to pharmacological therapy.

Chiropractic Therapy

The basic tenets of chiropractic therapy are controversial, but there is no question that this approach is enormously popular. Many patients use chiropractors in conjunction with physical therapy. They find chiropractic manipulation and massage beneficial for musculoskeletal pain and often for the neuropathic pain of GBS. They value the dietary and life style advice often given by chiropractors. With rare exceptions, no harm results. Vigorous cervical spinal manipulation has been associated with stroke and should be avoided.

Massage Therapy

Massage as a treatment for various ailments dates back 4,000 years, or more. It consists of manual (hand) techniques, including the application of pressure, holding, and movement of the body. Massage involves stroking, kneading, tapping compression, pressure, and rocking, which are applied to various parts of the body. These techniques are reported to affect the nervous and other systems of the body. The goal, according to an NIH review, is to "positively affect the health and well being of the client." Reported benefits include relief of sore muscles, increased flexibility and range of motion, decrease of chronic pain, and calming of the nervous system. There are several types of massage therapy, including neuromuscular massage, deep tissue massage, and hydrotherapy. Most states require licensing for this field. There is widespread interest in massage, but to what extent it can help GBS patients is unclear. Massage is also utilized by other disciplines, including occupational and physical therapy, without necessarily labeling their techniques as "massage therapy."

Hatha Yoga

The aim of this method of slow exercise, which originated in India, is to control and strengthen the body and mind and to reach a state of tranquility. It likely provides some measure of muscle strengthening and relaxation. It may offer a way to improve muscular function after GBS.

Vitamin, Mineral, and Herbal Supplements

Certain vitamins are essential for normal nerve function; however, dietary deficiency of these vitamins is extraordinarily rare in developed countries. An autoimmune disease of the stomach can prevent intestinal absorption of vitamin B^{12} from the diet, leading to a disease called *pernicious anemia.* Vitamin B^{12} deficiency resulting in this type of anemia can also cause damage to the spinal cord and possibly neuropathy. There is no evidence that providing supplementary vitamin B^{12} to individuals who do not have pernicious anemia is helpful in improving nerve regeneration. However, there is no known toxicity from B^{12}, so no harm can come from taking oral supplements of this vitamin.

Vitamin B^{6} *(pyridoxine)* is also needed for normal nerve function. This vitamin is widely available in the diet, and dietary deficiency is rare. Unlike most other vitamins, vitamin B^6 can be toxic to the nerves if taken in high doses, and should be limited to 20 mg daily. Multivitamin preparations usually contain only 5 mg of B^6, so these are safe. Check the label information carefully to determine how much vitamin B^6 a supplement contains in order to avoid any possibility of nerve damage.

Many different minerals have been touted as enhancing nerve regeneration, without scientific support. Mineral supplementation is considered harmless, but it has been shown that taking too much zinc can cause loss of copper from the body, leading to damage of the spinal cord. Herbal remedies and other nonprescription supplements, such as evening primrose oil and fish oils rich in omega-3 fatty acids, have their proponents and may actually have some health benefits, but any effect on nerve regeneration is unproven. The standard medical teaching is that a normal diet supplies sufficient vitamins and minerals for most people. Many GBS patients take supplements despite the lack of evidence as to benefit. Supplements are inexpensive and, for the most part, harmless.

Magnetic Therapy

Magnetized inserts placed into the shoes have been promoted to relieve pain. In one study, patients with neuropathic pain from diabetic neuropathy did appear to derive some benefit from this practice, but magnetic therapy must be considered unproven. The inserts are expensive, but harmless. Magnetic mattresses have also been promoted, but there is no evidence of benefit for any disorder. These mattresses are also harmless, but expensive.

Other complementary approaches include homeopathy, aromatherapy, reflexology, copper bracelets, hypnosis, transcendental meditation, and hydrotherapy, to name just a few. Evidence of benefit is lacking, but these practices are harmless. One major problem with alternative approaches is that the practitioners of these arts are often zealots for their cause and encourage their use as an alternative to conventional approaches. Use of these approaches as a complement to conventional therapy is seldom harmful, but stopping a medical therapy with proven benefit to adopt an alternative approach can carry significant risk. An open and honest discussion with your physician is strongly advised before embarking on one of these treatments.

ORGAN DONATION AND RECEIPT

Concern about organ donation and receipt occasionally arise. There are several reports of patients developing GBS following bone marrow transplantation (BMT), almost all associated with cytomegalovirus (CMV) infection, a well-recognized trigger for GBS. GBS can occur immediately following the transplant or many months later, indicating that it is not the procedure itself that triggers the GBS. GBS following solid organ transplantation is exceptionally rare. A recovered GBS patient is probably at no greater risk of developing GBS following BMT than an individual who has never had GBS. Furthermore, transplantation of any kind is done only in life-threatening situations, and the small risk of developing GBS must be weighed against the benefits of the transplant. BMT or solid organ transplantation should be considered only in extreme situations for a GBS patient still in the process of recovering. There is almost no situation in which the transplant could not be delayed until a more opportune time.

Fully recovered GBS patients can probably safely donate organs after death (cadaveric organ donation), although there is very little data on this to guide in making this decision. If a GBS patient has had particularly severe GBS, the possibility of organ damage during the acute illness must be considered. There is no recognized contraindication to a fully recovered GBS patient acting as a live organ donor, but recovering or incompletely recovered patients probably should not consider live organ donation.

The situation is different for patients with chronic inflammatory demyelinating polyneuropathy (CIDP) (see Chapter 9). Certainly they should not volunteer as live organ donors because the procedure of harvesting the organ may induce a relapse of their CIDP. It is completely unclear whether they can safely be considered as cadaveric organ donors, but they probably should not, particularly if their CIDP still required treatment at the time of death. There is probably no reason why a CIDP patient cannot be an organ or bone marrow recipient provided their CIDP is not severe and is well controlled. In fact, the immune suppression used to prevent transplant rejection is likely also to suppress the activity of CIDP.

CHAPTER 9

Chronic Immune-Mediated Polyneuropathies

Chronic acquired demyelinating neuropathies have many clinical, Celectrophysiologic (EMG), and pathological similarities to GBS, differing chiefly by virtue of the pace of progression. CIDP is the commonest of these disorders but all occur with less frequency than GBS. However, they are life-long conditions so that at any one time there are many more patients with these collective disorders than there are with GBS. They assume an even greater importance because, unlike most chronic neuropathies, they are treatable.

Four chronic immune-mediated polyneuropathies are discussed in this chapter: chronic inflammatory demyelinating polyneuropathy (CIDP), multifocal motor neuropathy (MMN), the Lewis-Sumner syndrome (multifocal, demyelinating motor and sensory neuropathy), and paraproteinemic neuropathy.

CHRONIC INFLAMMATORY DEMYELINATING POLYNEUROPATHY (CIDP)

What Is Chronic Inflammatory Demyelinating Polyradiculoneuropathy (CIDP) and How Does It Affect You?

CIDP, like Guillain-Barré syndrome (GBS), is an immune-mediated (autoimmune) disorder caused by the immune system attacking peripheral nerve myelin. It shares many clinical, electrophysiologic, and pathologic features with GBS. The main differences are the rate of evolution, prognosis, and, to some extent, the response to treatment. Indeed, 10 to 15 percent of cases of CIDP have an acute presentation virtually indistinguishable from GBS, and the initial attack may even resolve spontaneously and completely, only to relapse at a later date. Conversely, some degree of relapse during the recovery phase of GBS, although uncommon, does occur in about 5 percent of patients with otherwise typical disease and does not appear to predict progression to CIDP. Thus, it may be difficult at the time of the acute attack to be sure whether the disease is CIDP or GBS. It is important to recognize that having residual symptoms and signs from an attack of GBS is not the same as having CIDP. Many patients, as discussed in Chapter 8, may have symptoms of weakness, numbness, pain, or fatigue that may persist for years after recovery from an attack of GBS. However, these symptoms are not the result of continuing, immune attack on the peripheral nerve myelin; they simply represent incomplete regeneration of damage nerve fibers. Therefore, treatment of these patients with drugs such as intavenous immunogloulin (IVIg) or steroids is not indicated. The factors that determine the differences in the course of these two closely related autoimmune neuropathies are unknown.

The major difference between GBS and CIDP is the temporal profile of these diseases. In the majority of CIDP patients (about 75 percent), the disease develops over several months and progresses inexorably. Occasionally, the progression stabilizes without obvious deterioration for periods of weeks or months. About a quarter of the patients with CIDP have a relapsing course; that is, the disease occurs in attacks that may last weeks to months before improving, either spontaneously or with treatment, only to relapse again in the future. The relapsing form, in its first attack, closely resembles GBS, although the rate of deterioration is usually slower and bulbar and respiratory involvement is much less frequent, although they can occur. CIDP in children more closely resembles GBS, with patients progressing over a few months, stabilizing, and then improving over months. However, children, too, may have a slowly progressive down hill course over years.

The most prominent clinical feature of CIDP is weakness. It affects both proximal (closer to the body) and distal (farther away from the body) muscles early, but as the disease progresses, the distal muscle involvement becomes more noticeable. There is usually accompanying muscle atrophy. Patients may have muscle cramps and may notice twitching (fasciculations) in the muscles. Weakness of the bulbar muscles controlling speech and swallowing and other cranial muscles can occur but only on rare occasions. Similarly, weakness of the breathing muscles is occasionally encountered, although in contrast to GBS, mechanical ventilation is almost never necessary. Sensory functions are invariably affected in CIDP, more so than in GBS. While weakness occurs proximally and distally, numbness and tingling is confined to the distal limbs, seldom extending above the knees and elbows. Poor balance is also common because of involvement of sensory nerves that detect movements (proprioceptive nerves). Tremor may also occur when there is significant proprioceptive sensory loss. Reflexes are always diminished to some degree in CIDP, and usually they are completely absent. Neuropathic pain (see Chapter 8) is not common in CIDP, but it does occur more commonly than it does in GBS. Patients may complain of burning, stabbing, and shooting and aching pains in the feet and sometimes in the hands. The pain is usually worse at night and can lead to sleep disturbance. Fatigue is also common. Autonomic involvement can be found on careful testing in many CIDP patients but unlike GBS is rarely clinically significant.

How Is CIDP Diagnosed?

Physical Examination

The clinical features of CIDP resemble many other neuropathies and the disease cannot be reliably distinguished at the bedside. The clinical features that help separate CIDP from other chronic neuropathies are the predominance of weakness and the degree of reflex loss. Most other chronic neuropathies like diabetic neuropathy or toxic neuropathy have predominantly sensory features and reflex loss is confined to the ankle reflex.

Electrodiagnostic Testing

The most reliable way to diagnose CIDP is through electrodiagnostic testing (see Chapter 3 for details). Like GBS, CIDP is a demyelinating neuropathy so the essential features of the electrodiagnostic testing are very similar to those seen in GBS (see Chapter 3). The most characteristic feature is severe slowing of motor nerve conduction velocity. Conduction block and dispersion of the responses are also seen. Because of the chronic nature of the disease, there is usually progressive degeneration of the axons as well as demyelination, and as a result the amplitude of the responses produced by the electrical stimulation is reduced. As a result of this axonal degeneration, it can be difficult to identify the underlying demyelination;

once an axon has degenerated, it is impossible to tell what caused the degeneration. Thus, many different nerves and different nerve segments may need to be studied, explaining why the nerve conduction studies in CIDP may need to be so extensive. If multiple nerves and nerve segments are studied, the demyelinating nature of CIDP can be demonstrated in about 90 percent of cases.

Cerebrospinal fluid (CSF) Examination

Lumbar puncture does not always need to be done in patients with suspected CIDP. If the clinical picture is typical and the electromyogram (EMG) shows the expected changes of demyelination, the CSF examination is probably superfluous. However, if there are atypical features, particularly in cases where there is accompanying severe axonal degeneration, CSF examination may be useful. Once again, the abnormalities in the CSF in CIDP patients are essentially identical to those seen in GBS. The protein level is increased and there are no inflammatory cells, although patients who develop CIDP in association with human immunodeficiency virus (HIV) infection may have inflammatory cells.

Nerve Biopsy

Nerve biopsy is seldom necessary in CIDP, but in atypical cases it may be useful. As with the CSF examination, the cases that may need a biopsy are those in whom there is a lot of axonal degeneration. In CIDP, the nerve fibers may show thinning of the myelin sheath. In some cases, inflammation surrounding the small blood vessels in the nerve is also found. More often, nonspecific changes of axonal degeneration are found. Thus, it is important to recognize that having a nerve biopsy does not guarantee that a definite diagnosis can be reached.

Laboratory Testing

There are no blood or urine tests that can be done to make a diagnosis of CIDP. The purpose of laboratory testing is to make sure that there is not some other process occurring that could mimic CIDP (Table 9-1).

1. **Lyme disease:** On rare occasions, a neuropathy can be seen in patients with Lyme disease, so a blood test for antibodies to the Lyme organism should be done.
2. **Vasculitis:** When there is a lot of axonal degeneration, vasculitis (inflammation of the blood vessels) causing nerve damage can resemble CIDP, and blood tests for this may be requested.
3. **Paraproteinemic neuropathy:** As will be discussed below, a demyelinating neuropathy may occur in association with abnormal antibodies in the blood, a condition called paraproteinemic neuropathy. All patients with suspected CIDP should have a blood test called immunofixation in which the different antibody fractions in the blood can be measured. Many doctors also have blood tested for specific antibodies to different components of the nerve, called antiglycolipid

antibodies. Glycolipids are chemicals that are essential building blocks for the myelin, and on rare occasions a neuropathy is caused by antibodies to these chemicals. However, measuring these antibodies is unnecessary in the majority of cases of CIDP.

Table 9-1. Laboratory Testing in Pathients with CIDP

• Serum immunofixation: If a monoclonal protein is found, the patient should have a skeletal x-ray survey and a bone marrow examination.

• Serum Lyme test. If there is a high suspicion for Lyme disease, a CSF Lyme test may be done.

• Blood count, erythrocyte sedimentation rate (ESR), and antinuclear antibody (ANA) testing to assess for possible vasculitis.

What Causes CIDP?

We probably know less about the cause of CIDP than we do about the cause of GBS. CIDP is much less common than GBS and is not so well studied. CIDP is more common in men by an almost 2:1 ratio. CIDP affects all age groups, but the disease frequency increases with age, at least during the first six decades; very few cases with onset over the age of

70 years have been described. Like GBS, CIDP is a disease in which the nerve damage is caused by an abnormally directed immune response, but what actually triggers this abnormal response is unknown. It seems likely that the same factors that may lead to GBS could also lead to CIDP, but it is not known exactly why one is a monophasic illness that runs its course over a few months and then recovers, partly or completely, never to return and the other is chronic and probably life long.

It appears that development of CIDP requires both a genetic predisposition and an environmental factor. The environmental factors are unknown as no consistent culprit has been identified. Some studies have suggested a relationship to hepatitis vaccination but this remains unproven. There is no clear tie-in to any of the recognized triggers for GBS. Preceding events are identified in only 10 to 20 percent of patients, although in one study, 32 percent of patients had a preceding infection (the most commonly identified was cytomegalovirus) or vaccination. This is probably at least partly due to the chronicity of the disease; by the time the weakness becomes obvious, the patient has probably forgotten any illness that might have occurred immediately before the onset of the immune attack on the nerves. CIDP is more common in patients with HIV infection than would be expected from a chance association alone. Also,

CIDP is more likely to appear or relapse during pregnancy or immediately after delivery.

Although no definite trigger has been identified that leads to the development of CIDP, it does appear that concurrent infections and other illnesses may lead to relapses in the disease. This is usually manifested as increased weakness or sensory symptoms in someone who has been stable on treatment, necessitating an increase in the need for treatment. In some cases, the CIDP may be in remission and the patient on no chronic treatment and an event such as one of those noted above may precipitate reappearance or worsening of symptoms. If the CIDP is of the relapsing type, a relapse may be induced in the same way.

Vaccinations may rarely also cause a CIDP relapse. The medical advisory board of the GBS Support Group of the United Kingdom has addressed this matter and provided a series of recommendations that include:

1. Patients Not on Immunotherapy: These patients should receive vaccinations only if the benefit clearly outweighs the risk of precipitating a relapse.
2. Patients on Corticosteroids, Azathioprine, or other Immunosuppressive Drugs: These patients are less likely to have a relapse of CIDP because they are on immunosuppressive therapy, but that same therapy may increase their risk of developing an infection, such as

a serious case of the flu. In these patients, the benefit of vaccination may outweigh the risk.

3. Patients on Immunoglobulin (IVIg) Therapy: As a result of IVIg therapy, these patients are protected from infections. This decreases the need for vaccination. Also, IVIg may decrease the effectiveness of immunizations. If a patient elects to receive an immunization, it should be given half-way between two courses of IVIg therapy.

How Is CIDP Treated?

There are several treatments that have been proven to benefit patients with CIDP, and a number of others that may have an ancillary role. The proven treatments are corticosteroids, plasmapheresis, and high-dose intravenous immunoglobulin (IVIg). As well as treating the underlying abnormal immune response, treatment of the symptoms associated with CIDP is important.

Proven Treatments

Corticosteroids ("Steroids"). The most commonly used steroid is prednisone but others such as dexamethasone (Decadron) and methylprednisolone (Solu-Medrol or Medrol) are sometimes used. There is no evidence that one steroid is preferable to others. The steroids that we use to treat CIDP are not the same as the steroids that athletes sometimes use to strengthen their muscles to give them a competitive advantage. Most clinical trials of steroids in CIDP have used prednisone. Prednisone is given by mouth, usually on a daily or every other day basis. There is no question that it is a highly effective treatment. Steroids were first used for CIDP in the 1950s and there are many reports showing their effectiveness. Doctors at the Mayo Clinic, in the early 1980s, were the first to report the results of a careful scientific study proving the effectiveness of steroids in treating CIDP. More recently, steroids were compared to IVIg and the two treatments were found to be equally effective. The treatment is extremely inexpensive, and it is convenient for the patient since dosing is by mouth, whereas plasmapheresis and IVIg require intravenous treatment. Why, then, do we not treat everyone with steroids? The problem is the adverse effects. Steroids do not cure CIDP, they simply control the disease, and they usually have to be given in high doses for long periods of time. As a result, all patients receiving steroids experience side effects and some of them are serious (Table 9-2). It may be possible to reduce the frequency of administration to every other day so that the side effects are manageable. We have also experimented with even less frequent dosing, giving a very high dose once a week, and found it to be even safer, but its efficacy is unproven.

Plasmpheresis (Plasma exchange or PLEX). Since CIDP is an autoimmune disease in which antibodies to myelin attack the peripheral nerves, any strategy that removes antibodies from the circulation should have a beneficial effect on the disease. PLEX is such a strategy that has been shown to benefit patients with CIDP. The procedure is the same as for GBS (see Chapter 7). The procedure usually requires a high blood flow through the machine and therefore a large vein so a catheter may have to be implanted into the large veins around the shoulder. This is not much of a problem for GBS patients since the duration of the disease is short, but it is not a satisfactory solution for CIDP patients, who usually have to be treated for many years. The effect of PLEX is relatively short; most patients need to be retreated every few weeks for many years. Thus, PLEX is expensive and inconvenient. It is a useful strategy for the short-term management of CIDP but not for the necessary lifelong treatment. It does have the advantage that it is generally well tolerated. Some patients have a fall in blood pressure during the procedure but it is seldom serious. Repeated PLEX can lead to anemia and a low white blood cell count. If a long-term indwelling venous catheter is needed, it may become infected.

Table 9-2. Steroid Side Effects

Weight gain	Hair loss
Diabetes	Excessive facial hair (women)
Stomach ulcers (indigestion, heartburn)	Constipation or diarrhea
Bruising	Thin, fragile skin
Acne	Menstrual irregularity
Hypertension	Irritability*
Cataracts	Euphoria*
Fluid retention causing ankle swelling	Depression*

Muscle weakness	Insomnia*
Osteoporosis (thin bones) with risk of fractures	

* These side effects are much more common with high-dose "pulsed" steroids.

Intravenous Immunoglobulin (IVIg). IVIg has become the mainstay for the long-term treatment of CIDP. There have been several studies proving that IVIg improves CIDP patients better than placebo and that the treatment is just as effective as PLEX or steroids. Like these other treatments, IVIg is not a cure. It controls the disease but it does not make it go away. Thus, patients with CIDP need to be treated for years or decades and possibly for life. As the name (intravenous) implies, IVIg needs to be given by vein, but there are several advantages over PLEX. First, since the product is be infused into the veins without any blood needing to be removed, it can usually be given through a peripheral vein and usually does not require an indwelling venous catheter. However, because infusions have to be given frequently for very long periods of time, the peripheral veins may become very difficult to access, necessitating a central venous line eventually. Second, IVIg does not require an expensive machine to do the infusions so the treatment can be given at home. A nurse comes into the home to start the infusion and may need to stay throughout the infusion period of 2 to 4 hours, although in many cases, patients or family members can be trained to remove the needle once the infusion has finished. Medicare will not pay for home infusions so Medicare patients will need to be treated at an infusion center. It is this simplicity of administration that makes IVIg preferable to PLEX for long-term treatment of CIDP. However, there are disadvantages. The treatment is extremely expensive, both in terms of the cost of the product and the personnel costs associated with its administration, and insurance companies are often reluctant to allow continued treatment indefinitely. Significant adverse effects are uncommon but, when they do occur, can be serious (Table 9-3). Many patients experience headache during the infusion, although this is usually minor and improves once the infusion stops or even if the infusion rate is reduced. Acetominophen given prior to infusion and repeated as needed is usually sufficient to prevent the headache, and many patients do not want any treatment because the headache is so mild. Various allergic reactions can also occur (see Table 9-3) and diphenhydramine (Benadryl) is often given prior to infusion to prevent or minimize these. The most serious side effects are related to blood clots. IVIg infusion increases the likelihood of blood clots forming in the circulation. If these form in the veins, they can travel to the lungs, causing a condition called pulmonary embolism that can be fatal. If they form in the arteries, they can cause strokes or heart attacks. Kidney failure can also occur. Fortunately, blood clots are very rare but the risk does increase as the patient gets older. Also, the risk is increased if the patient is a smoker, has high blood cholesterol, has high blood pressure, diabetes, or heart disease, or has a family history of premature vascular disease. If any of these risk factors exist, IVIg needs to be used with caution. Reducing the infusion rate may reduce the risk of these complications, and it is probably not prudent to treat older patients or those with the listed risk factors at home.

Table 9-3. IVIg Side Effects

Headache (during infusion)
Chest tightness, breathlessness
Nausea, vomiting
Itching, rash
Blood clots leading to*:

- Heart attacks
- Strokes
- Pulmonary embolism (blood clots to the lungs)
- Kidney failure

Allergic meningitis (headache occurring after infusion)

*Treatment should be used with caution in patients already at risk for blood clots, including the elderly and those with diabetes, high blood pressure, or high cholesterol or a history of heart attack, stroke, or kidney disease.

Unproven Treatments

There are several other treatments that are used for CIDP whose benefits are unproven. However, there have been very few controlled studies, and clinical experience suggests that these drugs may have an important role. Treatment of CIDP with these agents should be confined to centers with considerable experience with their use

Azathioprine (Imuran), Methotrexate, and Mycophenylate Mofetil (Cellcept). These drugs are widely used, mainly in combination with one of the proven treatments rather than as sole therapy. These drugs are all immune suppressants; that is, they reduce the overactive immune response that is damaging the nerves. Azathioprine and mycophenylate are primarily used in transplant patients to prevent rejection of the transplanted organ, while methotrexate is mainly used to treat cancer. Methotrexate should always be given with folic acid because it reduces the activity of this essential vitamin. Each of these drugs can be used in combination with steroids, enabling the steroid dose to be reduced to less toxic levels. By combining two drugs with different side effects but additive beneficial effects, the desired therapeutic response may be obtained by using lower doses of each drug and minimizing side effects. For example, a patient on prednisone alone may require 20 to 40 mg a day, but the addition of azathioprine may enable the prednisone dose to be reduced to 20 mg every other day, a dose that may be largely free of serious adverse effects.

Cyclophosphamide. On rare occasions, more aggressive chemotherapy with cyclophosphamide (Cytoxan) may be tried. Once again, there are no studies that establish the effectiveness of this type of treatment. This treatment should only be given if everything else has failed since there are many side effects including hair loss, nausea and vomiting, liver toxicity, bone marrow toxicity, susceptibility to infection, and even a very small risk of subsequently developing leukemia or lymphoma and possibly bladder cancer.

Other Drugs. Several other drugs and drug combinations, such as *interferon-alpha, interferon-beta, rituximab,* and combined *PLEX/IVIg* have been tried, and continue to be studied in CIDP but must still be considered experimental.

Treatment of CIDP Symptoms

The common symptoms of CIDP that may need treatment independent of the treatment of the underlying disease are weakness, fatigue, and pain. Some patients have persistent footdrop despite best attempts to control the disease. Bracing with molded ankle-foot orthoses are important to help protect the patient against falls and ankle sprains or fractures. They may also help hip and back pain that can result from an abnormal gait related to footdrop. Persistent weakness in the hands may benefit from wrist support splints as well as outlined in Chapter 6.

Pain is a more common in CIDP than it is in GBS but, fortunately, is seldom severe. As with GBS, the pain may be neuropathic pain, due to nerve damage, or may be musculoskeletal, arising in joints and muscles, as a result of weakness. Neuropathic pain is generally felt on the surface of the skin and is burning, stinging, shooting, or stabbing in nature. It is most prominent in the feet and lower legs, rarely extending up as far as the knees. On occasion, it may occur in the hands. Neuropathic pain is usually worse at night and frequently disturbs the sleep. Some approaches to the treatment of neuropathic pain are outlined in Chapter 8. Musculoskeletal pain is generally felt in or around joints and is worse with weight bearing. It is relieved by rest and seldom disturbs sleep. It can be alleviated by appropriate bracing, and anti-inflammatory drugs such as naproxen, ibuprofen, or acetominophen may also help.

Fatigue is a very vexing symptom for CIDP patients and may occur even when there is not much weakness. There are no simple treatments. The principles of management of fatigue in CIDP are the same as in GBS, and are discussed in Chapter 8.

Prognosis in CIDP

CIDP is a long-standing disease that remains active for many years, whether it is in the form of periodic relapses or is chronically progressive. Complete recovery or long-term remission without any residual neurologic problems is achieved in less than 5 percent of patients. The other side of the coin is that very few patients die from CIDP or its complications. In their series of patients studied at the Mayo Clinic in the early 1970s, before the advent of effective treatment for the disease, Dr P. J. Dyck and his colleagues found that about 10 percent of patients died from the effects of the disease. In this series, two-thirds of the patients were treated with steroids but only for short periods of a few months' duration. Subsequent studies that included patients who had been treated more aggressively and for longer periods of time showed an even lower mortality (3 to 6 percent). Deaths mainly occur in the elderly and are usually from pulmonary (lung) complications such as pneumonia and pulmonary embolism (blood clots going to the lungs). Although death from CIDP is rare, few patients recover completely. Between 60 and 80 percent of patients are still able to work and function independently with minimal limitation. About 25 to30 percent have degrees of disability that range from being able to walk independently but unable to work to being confined to a wheelchair or to bed. Perhaps surprisingly, the patients with chronic progressive CIDP appear to do no worse than those with a relapsing course.

Case Study

A 42-year-old woman complained of tingling in her feet for 2 weeks followed by rapidly evolving weakness of arms and legs over 2 further weeks. Examination showed weakness in all limbs but no weakness in the face or throat and breathing functions were normal. All reflexes were absent. CSF protein was increased and electrodiagnostic studies showed demyelination. The patient was diagnosed with GBS, was treated with IVIg, and improved rapidly. At the time of her discharge from the hospital, she was able to walk without assistance and had only mild residual weakness. Six weeks later, she noted a return of her tingling and her weakness worsened. She again improved with IVIg treatment but relapsed within a few days after finishing the IVIg course. At this time, the diagnosis was changed to CIDP and she was treated with the corticosteroid medication methylprednisolone, with a good response. Her improvement has been maintained with intermittent doses of methylprednisolone.

MULTIFOCAL MOTOR NEUROPATHY (MMN) AND THE LEWIS-SUMNER SYNDROME

MMn

What is MMN and How Does It Affect You?

MMN is a curious chronic demyelinating neuropathy that differs from CIDP in two important respects. First, the demyelination is restricted to motor axons—those that control the muscles. Therefore, MMN patients have weakness but no numbness, tingling, or pain. Second, the demyelination is very patchy, affecting nerves in a seemingly random pattern and affecting only very short segments of the nerves. Therefore, the weakness only affects a few muscles. Like CIDP, this demyelination is thought to be immune mediated. The most obvious effect of this motor nerve demyelination is weakness, although the initial symptoms, at least in retrospect, may be muscle cramps or muscle twitching (called fasciculations). Most patients also develop muscle atrophy (wasting). The symptoms develop very slowly and usually progress over many years. Patients often do not seek medical advice until they have had the disease for 10 years or more. They may be completely unaware of muscle weakness in some areas and seek medical advice only when important functions, such hand function, are affected. One of my patients had virtually complete paralysis of the biceps muscle and had subconsciously developed trick movements to bend his elbow, and he remained completely unaware of that weakness until the hand became weak and he could no longer manipulate his nail clippers. Another curious feature is that the weakness is most often worse in the arms and hands, whereas most neuropathies, including CIDP, mainly affect the legs. The development of weakness, muscle atrophy, and fasciculations led to several patients with MMN being diagnosed with amyotrophic lateral sclerosis (Lou Gehrig's disease). Distinguishing MMN from Lou Gehrig's is critically important since MMN is a benign disease and is treatable, while Lou Gehrig's disease is always fatal and has no treatment. Peripheral nerves in patients may be enlarged enough to feel on clinical examination or enlargement can be seen with magnetic resonance imaging (MRI scan). On rare occasions, the enlargement may be so striking that it is thought to be a tumor. One of my patients developed a large swelling above the clavicle (collar bone) that was thought to be a tumor. The "tumor" was removed and found to be a hugely enlarged nerve. Similar nerve enlargement can be seen in CIDP but it is much less common.

How Is MMN Diagnosed?

Electrodiagnostic Testing (EMG)

As with CIDP, the diagnosis of MMN rests on the nerve conduction studies. When affected nerves are tested, severe or even complete block of electrical impulses is seen. Conduction velocity is severely slowed through that same segment of nerve. However, conduction velocity is completely normal along the rest of the nerve. Sensory nerve conduction studies are normal. These are important features that distinguish MMN from CIDP. In CIDP, there is more diffuse slowing of motor conduction velocity and sensory nerve conduction studies are usually abnormal.

Cerebrospinal Fluid (CSF) Examination

The CSF is normal in MMN, and spinal tap is not indicated unless there are very atypical features.

Nerve Biopsy

Since the sensory nerves are not involved in MMN and since it is unwise to biopsy motor nerves, nerve biopsy is not indicated in MMN.

Laboratory Testing

About half of all patients with MMN have very high levels of specific antibodies in their blood called anti-GM1 antibodies. They are directed against a specific component of the myelin sheath, the glycolipid. These antibodies can be measured in the blood. They do not need to be routinely measured unless there are unusual features and particularly if the patient appears clinically to have MMN, but does not have the expected abnormalities with the nerve conduction testing. There are no other useful laboratory tests.

What Causes MMN?

Like GBS and CIDP, MMN is an autoimmune disease. It is extremely rare, but the exact prevalence is not known. It affects men more than women. It is not known why only the motor nerves are affected. There is no recognized trigger for the disease, and there are no known associated diseases. The disease is more common in young people between 20 and 40 years of age, although children and the elderly are occasionally affected. Occasional periods of more rapid progression can be seen, but it is not clear that these are precipitated by any particular event.

How Is MMN Treated?

The only proven effective treatment for MMN is IVIg. Several studies have established the effectiveness of this treatment. However, IVIg does not cure the disease and long-term, probably life-long, treatment is necessary. The effect of the treatment usually lasts a few weeks to, at most, a few months. Most patients need to have the treatment repeated every 2 to 6 weeks. Cyclophosphamide may also help, but the risks usually outweigh the benefits. Patients may deteriorate more rapidly if treated with steroids or with PLEX.

Case Study

A 38-year-old man noticed painless wasting of the muscles in his right hand of 2 years' duration. He had noted no weakness, but weakness was found on examination. Sensation was normal. He had surgery to relieve a suspected entrapment of the nerve at his elbow, but there was no improvement. In fact, following the surgery, he developed weakness and fasciculations (muscle twitching) in the muscles of his thumb. The weakness interfered with his ability to work with his computer keyboard. At this time, he was thought have amyotrophic lateral sclerosis (Lou Gehrig's disease) and was sent for neurologic evaluation. Examination showed severe weakness of all the hand muscles with irregular twitching of the muscles. All other muscles were normal. Electrodiagnostic studies showed severe conduction block in the forearm nerves. Sensory studies were normal. Blood testing for GM1 antibodies showed very high levels. He was treated with a 5-day course of IVIg. Strength in the thumb muscles returned to normal, but he had mild residual weakness in the other hand muscles. He was able to return to his work without limitation. Three months later, the weakness returned to a mild degree and retreatment again resulted in improvement. He has continued to receive intermittent IVIg treatment every 3 to 4 months and maintains normal function.

Lewis-Sumner Syndrome

What Is the Lewis-Sumner Syndrome, How Does It Affect You and How Does It Differ from MMN?

In many ways, the Lewis-Sumner syndrome is similar to MMN. It is a slowly evolving, multifocal, demyelinating neuropathy. The only difference is that it affects both sensory and motor axons. Weakness is the most prominent feature of the disease, but patients also have loss of sensation and paresthesias (tingling, pins and needles) and occasionally neuropathic pain. Like MMN, the disease affects the arms more than the legs and is very patchy, affecting one or two nerves severely, while completely sparing adjacent nerves. Nerve conduction studies show the same motor conduction block and severe slowing of the transmission of the electrical stimuli. However, the sensory responses from the affected nerves are lost. Like MMN patients, the CSF is usually normal in Lewis-Sumner syndrome, although in a few patients, the protein level is increased. However, spinal tap is not necessary in most cases. The same antiglycolipid antibodies that are seen in about half the MMN patients may also be seen in Lewis-Sumner syndrome but they are less common. Treatment of Lewis-Sumner syndrome is the same as treatment of MMN. Thus, there are many more similarities between MMN and Lewis-Sumner syndrome than there are differences, and in my opinion, they are different facets of the same disease.

PARAPROTEINEMIC NEUROPATHY

What Is a paraproteinemic Neuropathy?

Another chronic demyelinating neuropathy that can resemble CIDP is *paraproteinemic neuropathy.* A paraprotein, also called a monoclonal protein, is an abnormal antibody in the blood that can occasionally attack the myelin of the peripheral nerves. Most commonly, we do not know the significance of the paraprotein, so we call the condition monoclonal gammopathy of undetermined significance (MGUS). Occasionally, the paraprotein is produced by a type of bone marrow cancer. Therefore, any patient who has a paraprotein must be carefully evaluated to exclude bone marrow cancer. This usually entails taking x-rays of multiple bones and doing a bone marrow biopsy. MGUS is not an uncommon condition;

about 6 to10 percent of the population over the age of 60 years has MGUS. It is possible that in many cases the association between demyelinating neuropathy and a paraprotein is no more than coincidental.

How Does a Paraproteinemic Neuropathy Affect You?

The clinical appearance of a typical paraproteinemic neuropathy is different from CIDP. Paraproteinemic neuropathy is a predominantly sensory disorder. The major complaints are numbness and tingling in the feet along with loss of balance that is often the most disabling feature. The imbalance is caused by degeneration of the nerve fibers called proprioceptive fibers that tell the brain where the limbs and body are in relationship to each other. The imbalance that results from proprioceptive sensory loss is different from other forms of loss of balance in that it is only present, or is at least much worse, in the dark or when the eyes are closed. Patients will often describe a tendency to fall over when they close their eyes in the shower or a tendency to stagger when they go to the bathroom in the night. When it is particularly bad, patients may be completely unaware of where their feet are without looking at them. One patient could not locate the foot controls of his car without looking under the dashboard. To make matters worse, he could not feel how hard he was pushing on the pedals, so his driving was very unsafe and his driving privileges had to be suspended. Typically, numbness and tingling begin in a symmetrical pattern involving the toes first and then spreading to the feet and lower legs. Hands are occasionally involved but never in the early stages. Neuropathic pain is uncommon but can occur. This prominent sensory loss is unusual in CIDP, which is predominantly a motor disorder. Weakness does occur in paraproteinemic neuropathy but it is a late feature. Furthermore, unlike CIDP, which usually has both proximal and distal weakness, the weakness in paraproteinemic neuropathy is restricted to the distal muscles. Paraproteinemic neuropathy is a disorder that progresses extremely slowly. Patients are often unable to clearly identify the onset of their symptoms and worsening occurs over decades. This is in contrast to CIDP, which typically progresses over months to a year or two. Paraproteinemic neuropathy is very much a disorder of the elderly; the majority of patients are over the age of 70, contrasting with CIDP, which can occur at any age but tends to be focused on people in mid life. Thus, paraproteinemic neuropathy is a predominantly sensory, indolently progressive disorder of older patients, whereas CIDP is a predominantly motor disorder that is subacutely progressive and affects younger patients. The differences between these two demyelinating neuropathies are summarized in Table 9-4. It is important to emphasize that none of these differences allows an absolute clinical distinction to be made between them. However, patients with paraproteinemia never have a neuropathy that could be mistaken for typical CIDP, whereas patients with CIDP may be atypical and may have a clinical appearance that resembles the neuropathy seen with paraproteinemia.

Table 9-4. Differences Between CIDP and Paraproteinemic Neuropathy

CIDP	Paraproteinemic neuropathy
Predominantly motor	Predominantly sensory
Proximal and distal weakness	Strictly distal weakness
Diffuse loss of reflexes	Distal loss of reflexes
Subacute evolution (months to years)	Very chronic evolution (years to decades)
Any age	Elderly (usually over 70 years)
Patchy but widespread conduction slowing	Predominantly distal slowing
CSF protein usually elevated	CSF protein usually normal

How Is Paraproteinemic Neuropathy Diagnosed?

Electrodiagnostic Testing

Like CIDP, paraproteinemic neuropathy is usually a demyelinating disorder, but the distribution of the demyelination differs in the two conditions. In CIDP, the demyelination, and therefore the slowing of the speed of conduction, is in a patchy distribution and is seen in both proximal and distal nerve segments. In paraproteinemic neuropathy, the conduction slowing is usually confined to the most distal segments at the onset of the disease, resulting in marked prolongation of the time for the impulses to travel the last few centimeters to the muscle. As the disease progresses, the conduction slowing moves up the nerves. Conduction block is rarely seen in paraproteinemic neuropathy. If this pattern of strictly distal slowing without conduction block is not present, it is more likely that the presence of the paraprotein is a coincidence and that the patient has CIDP and is more likely to respond to treatment.

Cerebrospinal Fluid Examination

The CSF is usually normal in paraproteinemic neuropathy.

Nerve Biopsy

The nerve biopsy shows thinning of the myelin sheath, as in other demyelinating neuropathies. In some forms of paraproteinemic neuropathy, there is a highly characteristic appearance of the myelin that can help establish the diagnosis. Inflammation should not be present in paraproteinemic neuropathy.

Laboratory Testing

All patients with acquired demyelinating neuropathy should be tested for the presence of a paraprotein. This can be done with a blood test called electrophoresis, but this test picks up only about 85 percent of paraproteins, so it is recommended that the more sensitive test called immunofixation should be done.

If a paraprotein of any kind is found, regardless of its relationship to the associated neuropathy, a meticulous search for an underlying malignancy must be made. This may identify a cancer of the bone marrow, such as multiple myeloma, or a solitary tumor called a plasmacytoma. Bone marrow examination and a regular x-ray of bones of the spine and around the hips and shoulders should be done.

How Is Paraproteinemic Neuropathy Treated?

1. If the paraproteinemic neuropathy is associated with underlying malignancy, treatment is with chemotherapy, aimed at eliminating the cancer. If the cancer can be eliminated, the paraprotein disappears and the neuropathy stabilizes and there may be partial improvement, although complete return to normal is unlikely.
2. If the paraproteinemic neuropathy is associated with a solitary plasmacytoma, treatment may be radiation therapy to the area of the tumor or surgical excision of the tumor if it is accessible. The solitary plasmacytoma can usually be totally eliminated and, as a result, the paraprotein disappears and the neuropathy resolves or improves. This is the form of paraproteinemic neuropathy that has the best prognosis.

Case study: A 34-year-old man presented with distal leg weakness that progressed over 6 months. He had tingling sensations in his toes and a sense of numbness on the soles of his feet. The upper limbs were not involved. EMG studies showed a mainly demyelinating neuropathy. Serum immunofixation showed a paraprotein. Spinal x-rays showed a single bony tumor in the spine, and a biopsy of the tumor showed it to be a plasmacytoma. Because of the location of the tumor, complete surgical excision was not thought to be possible so the tumor was irradiated. Following radiation the strength rapidly returned to normal. Two years later, there has been no recurrence of the tumor and the strength remains normal.

3. If the paraprotein is related to MGUS, treatment is not imperative since the underlying condition is relatively benign. However, the neuropathy may be disabling and treatment could be justified by virtue of the neuropathy itself. However, this type of neuropathy is very difficult to treat, and the risks of treatment must be weighed against the benefits. IVIg occasionally helps, but usually the treatment is some form of chemotherapy The most commonly used drugs are cyclophosphamide (Cytoxan) and chlorambucil (Leukeran). A newer form of chemotherapy with a drug called rituximab (Rituxan), which eliminates the antibody-forming cells, has been reported to be successful

in some cases. This treatment has the advantage that it is much better tolerated than traditional chemotherapy and only has to be administered for a short period of time.

Case study: A 78-year-old man presented with loss of balance and numbness in his feet that had slowly progressed over more than 5 years. His imbalance was much worse in the dark and he had to sit down in the shower to avoid falls. He had no complaints of weakness, but examination did show mild weakness confined to the feet. Electrodiagnostic studies showed a demyelinating neuropathy with marked accentuation of conduction slowing in the most distal segments of the nerves. Serum immunofixation showed an IgM paraprotein with antibodies to MAG. He wished to be treated and chlorambucil was started. There was very slow improvement over the following 2 years, so that he went from using a wheelchair most of the time to walking with a walker and then with a cane and he was able to shower standing up. He became intolerant of the medication and it was stopped. There was a slow decline in function so that he needed the walker again after about a year and became wheelchair dependent again after 2 years.

The chronic, acquired demyelinating neuropathies are immunemediated disorders that are uncommon but important causes of disability. They are distinguished from GBS primarily by their chronic course, which evolves over months to years, although CIDP occasionally has an acute onset that is initially indistinguishable from GBS. The importance of these disorders is greater than their relative rarity suggests because, in contrast to many chronic neuropathies, they may benefit from treatment, thereby minimizing that disability.

Glossary

Achilles tendon: The tendon at the back of the ankle. A doctor may hit this tendon with a hammer to elicit a reflex in patients with GBS or CIDP.

Acidosis: The condition that results in the accumulation of metabolic acids in the blood.

Active range of motion exercise: An exercise, performed by a patient, in which a joint is moved through its maximal range using the patient's own muscle strength.

Activities of daily living (ADL): The usual activities carried out during normal daily life. Such activities include walking, climbing stairs, personal hygiene (bathing, toileting, brushing teeth, combing hair), dressing, and others.

Acute: Rapidly progressive. In the context of neuropathy, this indicates a condition that evolves over days to weeks.

Acute infectious polyneuritis: An old name for GBS. It is a misnomer since there is no infection of the nerve.

Acute inflammatory demyelinating polyneuropathy (AIDP): The most common form of GBS that primarily damages the myelin sheath.

Acute motor axonal neuropathy (AMAN): The most common form of axonal GBS in which the axonal damage is restricted to the motor axons.

Acute motor and sensory axonal neuropathy (AMSAN): A less common and more severe form of axonal GBS in which the axonal damage affects both motor and sensory nerve fibers.

Aerobic training: A form of exercise that increases the ability of the muscles to use oxygen to generate energy. Examples of aerobic exercise include walking, bicycling, swimming, and running.

Ambu bag: A compressible, air-filled bag that can be connected to a face mask or endotracheal tube that allows a patient to be ventilated by hand.

Ambulation: Walking.

Amyotrophic lateral sclerosis (ALS): A fatal disease of the motor nerves, also known as Lou Gehrig's disease.

Analgesics: Medications used to treat pain.

Anterior: The front of the body.

Anticoagulants: Medications that prevent thrombosis (blood clots).

Antigen: A chemical, usually a protein, which stimulates the immune system to produce antibodies.

Anti-glycolipid antibodies: Antibodies that attack a group of chemicals that contain glucose (glyco-) and fat (lipid), that are an important component of the nerve fiber.

Areflexia: Loss of the reflexes that are elicited during a neurological examination by tapping the tendon of a muscle with a rubber hammer.

Arrhythmia: Irregular or abnormal heart beat.

Arterial blood gas (ABG): A test that measures blood levels of oxygen and carbon dioxide.

Aspiration: Descent of material, such as food or liquid, down the airway into the lungs.

Aspiration pneumonia: Pneumonia caused by aspiration of food into the lungs.

Ataxia: A condition in which there is loss of co-ordination and balance.

Atelectasis: Collapse of small segments of the lung. Atelecatasis is common in GBS patients and may be an antecedent to pneumonia.

Autonomic nervous system (ANS): That part of the nervous system that automatically controls internal organs of the body. Examples of organs and functions controlled by the ANS include the heart, blood pressure, heart rate, bladder activity, and bowel motility.

Autoimmune: A condition in which the immune system attacks some component of the body. In GBS and CIDP the immune system attacks peripheral nerves.

Axon: The part of the nerve that transmits electrical impulses.

Axonal Guillain-Barre syndrome: A form of GBS that primarily affects the axon.

Axonal neuropathy: Any peripheral neuropathy caused by damage to the axon.

Azathioprine (Imuran): A medication that suppresses the activity of the immune system and is used in the treatment of auto-immune diseases.

Bed mobility: The ability of a patient to move in bed. A normal person can readily move about in bed but if some muscles are too weak, as in severely affected GBS patients with weak back and limb muscles, independent movement in bed may be limited.

Bell's palsy: An acute neurological disorder that results in paralysis of the muscles of one side of the face.

Blood pressure: The pressure of the blood that is flowing in the circulation. The pressure is in part generated by influences of the heart beat, volume of blood in the circulation, and other factors.

Bradycardia: Slow heart rate.

Brain-derived neurotrophic factor: A chemical produced in the brain that supports and stimulates nerve growth.

Bronchodilator: A drug that causes widening of the bronchi (air passages), thereby making it easier to breathe, usually given to patients with asthma or chronic bronchitis.

Bulbar: Pertaining to the bulb, the lowest part of the brain called the medulla oblongata. The nerves that come from this part of the brain supply the muscles that control speech and swallowing.

Bulbar palsy: Weakness of muscles supplied by the bulbar nerves.

Campylobacter jejuni: A bacterium that is one of the most common causes of gastroenteritis and also one of the commonest infections that can trigger GBS.

Carbon dioxide (CO_2): The gas that is produced by the body's metabolism and that is excreted through the lungs during expiration.

; **Carbon dioxide narcosis:** Mental confusion that results from accumulation of carbon dioxide in the body.

Carpal tunnel syndrome: A condition of pain and paresthesias caused by entrapment of the median nerve in a tunnel formed by bones and ligaments at the wrist.

Cellcept: *See* mycophenylate mofetil.

Central nervous system: The part of the nervous system comprised of the brain and spinal cord.

Cerebrospinal fluid (CSF): A clear liquid that bathes the brain and spinal cord. The protein concentration in the CSF is increased in GBS and CIDP.

Chronic: Slowly progressive and long-lasting. In the context of neuropathy, this indicates a condition that evolves over months or years.

Chronic bronchitis: An inflammatory condition of the bronchi, the tubes that carry air from the trachea to the lungs. When the bronchi become inflamed, excessive secretions are generated and this may compromise air flow leading to breathlessness. Chronic bronchitis is most often caused by smoking.

Chronic inflammatory demyelinating polyneuropathy (CIDP): A chronic neuropathy that shares many characteristics with GBS. It differs primarily by virtue of its much slower evolution.

Chronic obstructive pulmonary disease (COPD): Two disorders, chronic bronchitis and emphysema, in which the lungs are irreversibly damaged. COPD is most often caused by smoking.

Clitoris: A female sexual organ.

Clavicle: Collar bone. The clavicles are the prominent bones on each side at the bottom of the neck.

Communication Cards: A set of cards that shows, in large print, a series of questions often asked by GBS patients. It is used for patients on ventilators, who cannot talk, to help them communicate with caregivers and visitors. It is available through the GBS/CIDP Foundation.

Contracture: Shortening of muscles, tendons, ligaments, and joint tissues that result in limited ability for a limb to be moved through its normal range of motion. For example, if the Achilles tendon at the lower end of the calf becomes shortened, the patient can not fully raise the front of the foot and is forced to walk on their toes.

Cornea: The clear structure that covers the front of the eye. Light passes through the cornea and registers images on the back of the eye (the retina) that are transmitted to the brain for interpretation.

Corticosteroids: Chemicals produced by the body but also manufactured for the treatment of inflammatory illnesses. They should not be confused with anabolic steroids that are sometimes used by athletes to build up muscle mass.

Cranial: Pertaining to the skull.

Cyclo-oxygenase inhibitors (see NSAIDS): A class of non-steroidal anti-inflammatory drug whose actions are the result of their ability to inhibit a specific enzyme called cyclo-oxygenase that is involved in inflammation.

Cyclophosphamide: A medication used in chemotherapy for the treatment of cancer. It is occasionally used to suppress the activity of the immune system for the treatment of auto-immune diseases.

Cytomegalovirus (CMV): A virus that commonly causes respiratory infections and that can trigger GBS.

Day hospital: A hospital that provides medical care and the site of care to a patient who has been discharged from a hospital to live at home but continues to need full-time care in the hospital setting during the day. A day hospital allows patients to live in the comfort of their home while still receiving a high level of rehabilitation and nursing care.

Decubiti: Breakdown of the skin caused by pressure, leading to ulceration.

Deep tendon reflexes: *See* muscle stretch reflexes.

Demyelinating neuropathy: A peripheral neuropathy caused by damage to the myelin sheath surrounding nerve fibers (axons).

Denervation: The loss of nerve supply to a part of the body.

Diaphragm: The major muscle of respiration located under the lungs and attached to the lower part of the rib cage. When the diaphragm contracts, air is sucked into the lungs.

Diastolic blood pressure: The pressure in the arteries recorded when the heart muscle is relaxed. This is the bottom number of the two numbers recorded when the blood pressure is measured.

Diplopia: Double vision.

Distal: Structures of the body most distant from the brain and spinal cord.

Doppler flow analysis: A non-invasive technique that can be used to detect blood flowing in the veins. If a patient has developed blood clots (venous thrombosis) the blood flow will be impeded and the Doppler flow analysis will enable accurate detection of the clots.

Dorsiflexion: Raising the front of the foot up by bending at the ankle.

Duplex study: Doppler flow analysis combined with ultrasound imaging of the veins to detect the presence of blood clots.

Durable medical equipment: Equipment such as wheelchairs or walkers that can be reused for long periods.

Dysrhythmia: *See* arrhythmia.

Edema: Swelling due to accumulation of fluid in the tissues.

Electromyography (EMG): A procedure in which the electrical activity of nerves and muscles can be recorded and analyzed to assess their state of health.

Emphysema: One of two common lung disorders, together called chronic obstructive pulmonary disease or COPD. The lungs contain innumerable small air sacs, called alveoli, where oxygen passes from the lungs into the blood and CO2 passes from the blood into the lungs. In emphysema the alveoli are permanently damaged, resulting in poor lung function and breathing.

Encephalitis: Inflammation of the brain which can cause headache, mental confusion, and seizures. It is usually caused by a viral infection.

Encephalomyelitis: Inflammation of the brain and spinal cord.

Encephalopathy: Mental confusion and sleepiness typically caused by accumulation of toxic chemicals in the brain. In GBS it can result from lack of oxygen, accumulation of carbon dioxide, medications, or abnormalities of blood chemistry.

Endotracheal tube: A flexible plastic tube that is inserted through the mouth or nose into the upper airway or trachea, to create a reliable means to provide artificial or mechanical breathing. It may also be used to protect the lungs from aspiration in patients with bulbar palsy.

Enzymes: A group of molecules in the body that enable the chemical reactions necessary for metabolism to occur. Enzymes are catalysts, molecules that enable chemical reactions to occur rapidly.

Epstein-Barr virus: The virus that causes infectious mononucleosis "mono" and that can also trigger GBS.

Erythema: An excessive red or pink discoloration of the skin. It may be a precursor to skin break-down and therefore, is an important sign to seek in patients who are immobile.

Expectorants: Medications given to make it easier to cough out secretions from the lungs.

Expiration: The act of breathing air out of the lungs.

Expiratory flow rate: The speed at which air flows out of the lungs when a person forcibly exhales. This is a measure of breathing or lung function.

Extubation: Removal of a tube. In GBS, this refers to removal the endotracheal tube from the trachea when a patient is ready to breathe on his own.

Fasciculation: Twitching of the muscles due to nerve damage.

Fibrillation: The electrical response recorded during the EMG procedure when a muscle fiber spontaneously activates. It is an indication of nerve damage.

Forced vital capacity: *See* vital capacity.

Formication: A form of paresthesia consisting of a sense of ants or other insects crawling under the skin.

Functional Independence measure instrument (FIMI): A method to measure and tabulate neuromuscular function. A record of a patient's functional ability can be used to identify rehabilitation gains and deficiencies so that therapists can plan specific exercises to address deficiencies.

Gastroenteritis: Inflammation of the bowel leading to nausea, vomiting and diarrhea, usually the result of food poisoning.

GBS/CIDP Foundation International: The Guillain-Barré Syndrome/Chronic Inflammatory Demyelinating Polyneuropathy Foundation International. Its foremost goal is support of GBS and CIDP patients and their loved ones.

Gycosylated hemoglobin: A form of hemoglobin with sugar molecules attached. It is increased in patients with diabetes and is measured as a way of monitoring the effectiveness of diabetes control.

Heart rate: The number of contractions of the heart that occurs each minute. The normal range is from 60 to 100 times a minute.

Heparin: A type of anticoagulant that is given by injection.

High resistance exercise: An exercise done to strengthen muscles. This is usually performed in a GBS patient when some use of a limb has returned, to increase strength.

Hyperalbuminosis: A medical term used by Dr. G. Guillain and his colleagues to describe the increased protein concentration in the cerebrospinal fluid.

Hypertension: Abnormally high blood pressure.

Hypotension: Abnormally low blood pressure.

Hypothyroidism: A condition resulting from insufficient thyroid hormone.

Immunoglobulin: The proteins in the blood plasma that contain the antibodies that are thought to attack the nerves in GBS. Immunoglobulin from donated blood is also administered intravenously to treat GBS and CIDP.

Immunofixation: A blood test that measures the concentration of immune proteins (antibodies) in the blood.

Impotence: Inability of the male to engage in sexual intercourse.

Imuran: *See* azathioprine.

Inferior vena cava: The large vein that drains the blood from the lower part of the body into the heart.

Innervation: The supply of nerves to a part of the body.

Insensible loss: Loss of fluids from the body by sweating and through the lungs. This contrasts with the loss of fluids that can be directly measured by recording urine output. Insensible loss of fluids is increased in patients with fever or with rapid respiratory (breathing) rate as may occur in GBS.

Inspiration: The act of breathing air into the lungs.

Inspiratory force: The pressure or suction that a patient can generate to breathe in. It is a measure of breathing or lung function. This test helps to measure the strength of the breathing muscles.

Intensive care unit (ICU): A section of a hospital designed to provide continuous surveillance and care to severely ill patients. The ratio of patients to nurses is small, with each nurse taking care of only 2 or 3 patients. ICU's also continuously monitor the heart beat, blood pressure, breathing rate, and oxygen concentration in the blood. Patients who require mechanical support of breathing are almost always in an ICU.

Intercostal muscles: The muscles located between the ribs. When the intercostal muscles contract, the front of the ribs are raised up and forward to expand the chest, enlarge the chest cavity, and expand the lungs. These muscles assist the diaphragm during inspiration (breathing in).

Intermittent mandatory ventilation (IMV): A technique used during weaning from a ventilator. The ventilator is set to deliver a predetermined minimum number of breaths every minute. If the patient has a breathing rate that is too slow, the ventilator will intermittently deliver a mandatory breath. This ensures that the patient continues to get adequate oxygen during the weaning process.

International normalized ratio: A standardized ratio that compares the clotting time of a patient to a normal standard that is used to monitor the effectiveness of anticoagulation.

Intubation: Insertion of a tube. Usually refering to the insertion of a tube through the nose or mouth into the trachea to enable breathing to be supported.

I/O chart: The chart that is maintained by the nursing staff that records all fluids that are taken in or passed out by the patient.

Laryngoscope: An instrument that enable the physician to look down into the larynx (voice box).

Larynx: Voice box.

Libido: Sexual drive or desire.

Locked-in syndrome: A condition in which the patient remains completely alert and aware of the surroundings but cannot communicate through speech or gestures because of paralysis of all muscles.

Low resistance exercise: An exercise done repeatedly and with little resistance with the goal of increasing stamina rather than strength.

Lumbar puncture: The procedure whereby a needle is inserted into the lower spine and cerebrospinal is fluid withdrawn for analysis.

Luteinizing hormone (LH): A hormone or chemical secreted by the pituitary gland at the base of the brain. LH is required for the testicles to maintain a normal blood level of testosterone. The finding in the blood of a decreased testosterone level and an elevated LH level will reflect the brain's attempt to compensate for the testosterone deficiency by making more LH.

Lyme disease: A condition that results from infection with the organism, *Borrelia burgdorferi,* contained in the saliva of the deer tick. It causes arthritis and a skin rash and may rarely affect the nerves.

Lymphocytes: White blood cells that carry out the functions of the immune system.

Macrophage: A cell that engulfs and destroys damaged tissue.

Mechanical ventilation: The process of providing breathing to a patient by a mechanical ventilator. This sophisticated medical device delivers air into the lungs through a plastic tube inserted into the patients airway.

Mechanical ventilator: *See* ventilator.

Methotrexate: A medication that suppresses the activity of the immune system and is used in the treatment of auto-immune diseases.

Miller Fisher syndrome: An unusual form of GBS that causes paralysis of eye muscles (ophthalmoplegia), loss of coordination and imbalance (ataxia), and loss of the tendon reflexes (areflexia).

Molded ankle-foot orthosis (MAFO): A device typically made of thin, light-weight plastic that fits under the foot and around the back of the leg and is used to compensate for foot drop.

Mononucleosis: An increase in a certain type of white blood cells in the circulation.

Motor: Pertaining to the control of muscles.

Muscle atrophy: Thinning of the muscle, usually due to damage to its nerve supply. Atrophy can also occur with disuse in someone confined to bed.

Muscle stretch reflexes: The involuntary contraction of a muscle in response to the tendon being tapped with a rubber hammer.

Mycophenylate mofetil (Cellcept): A medication that suppresses the activity of the immune system and is used in the treatment of autoimmune diseases.

Mycoplasma pneumoniae: A common organism that causes pneumonia and can also trigger GBS.

Myelin: The insulating layer that wraps around each axon in peripheral nerves and the central nervous system.

Nasal cannula: A plastic tube that can be inserted into the nose to deliver oxygen.

Nasogastric tube: A plastic tube that is passed through the nose into the stomach. It can be used for feeding or for withdrawing substances from the stomach.

Nerve conduction studies: A method of evaluating the function of peripheral nerves by electrically stimulating the nerves and recording the electrical responses of the nerves.

Nerve roots: The part of the peripheral nervous system that first emerges from the spinal cord.

Neuropathic: Pertaining to neuropathy.

Neuropathic pain: Pain resulting from damage to nerves.

Nociceptive: The normal ability to feel pain.

Nociceptive pain: Pain resulting from a noxious stimulus.

Nodes of Ranvier: The small gaps that are found between segments of myelin along the length of the nerve where electrical current is generated and renewed.

Non-steroidal anti-inflammatory drugs (NSAIDS): Drugs not related to steroids that are used to treat inflammation. They include aspirin, acetaminophen (Tylenol), ibuprofen, and naproxen among many others.

Occupational therapist: A medical professional who is trained to use exercise and other physical methods of treatment to assist patients to improve neuromuscular function so they can perform activities of daily living, such as dressing, grooming, cooking, and vocational activities.

Occupational therapy: A form of treatment that uses exercise and other physical methods of therapy to improve neuromuscular function.

Olfactory: Pertaining to the sense of smell.

Ophthalmoplegia: Paralysis or weakness of the muscles that control the movements of the eyes. Ophthalmoplegia usually causes double vision (diplopia) and drooping eyelids (ptosis).

Optic nerve: The nerve that conveys visual messages from the eye to the brain.

Optic neuritis: Inflammation of the optic nerve.

Orthostatic hypotension: A drop in blood pressure that occurs with standing.

Orthotic: A medical device that is attached externally to the body to improve or correct a deformity or improve a function of a movable part.

Paralytic ileus: Paralysis of the muscles of the bowel leading to severe constipation.

Papilledema: Swelling of the optic nerve.

Paraprotein: An abnormal protein in the blood produced by the immune cells.

Paraproteinemic neuropathy: A neuropathy resembling CIDP that results from a paraprotein attacking the nerve.

Parasympathetic nervous system: The part of the autonomic nervous system that primarily controls bowel and bladder function.

Paresthesias: Spontaneous, non-painful abnormal sensations, usually described as tingling or pins and needles.

Passive range of motion exercise: An exercise, performed on a patient by another person such as a therapist, in which a joint is moved through a maximal range of movement while the patient is fully relaxed.

PEG tube: The plastic tube that is passed through the gastrostomy opening into the stomach.

Percutaneous gastrostomy: The procedure whereby an opening is created through the abdominal wall into the stomach for the purpose of feeding.

Peripheral nervous system: The part of the nervous system comprised of the nerves that extend into the head, neck, torso, and limbs.

Peripheral neuropathy: Any abnormal condition affecting peripheral nerves.

Pernicious anemia: A form of anemia that results from a lack of vitamin B^{12}.

Peroneal: The area in the front of the leg, below the knee.

Pharynx: The area at the back of the throat where the mouth joins the esophagus.

Phlebitis: Inflammation of the veins, usually leading to blood clots.

Physiatrist: A doctor of medicine or osteopathy who specializes in physical medicine and rehabilitation.

Physiatry: The medical specialty of physical medicine and rehabilitation.

Physical therapist: A medical professional who is trained to administer

physical therapy or rehabilitation care.

Physical therapy: A form of treatment that uses exercise and other physical methods of therapy to assist a patient in improving neuromuscular function. Physical therapy is helpful to persons with physical disabilities, such as GBS.

Plantar flexion: Movement of the foot down. Pushing the front of the foot down is required as part of the initial 'push off' phase of walking.

Plasmapheresis (PLEX, plasma exchange): A form of treatment for GBS whereby the plasma portion of the blood is separated from the red and white blood cells and is discarded and replaced with plasma obtained from a blood donor.

Pneumothorax: Partial or total collapse of a lung that can occur if air enters the extremely small space, called the pleural space, between the inside of the chest wall and the lungs.

Posterior: The back of the body.

Post-herpetic neuralgia: A painful condition that occurs following an episode of shingles.

Post-polio syndrome: A condition resulting in pain and weakness that develops in individuals who have had polio many decades previously.

Postural hypotension: *See* orthostatic hypotension.

PRN: Pro re nata. This Latin term means when necessary or as warranted by the situation. It is often used to describe directions for using medication : e.g., take 2 aspirin every 4–6 hours prn (as needed for) pain, or to provide nursing directions : provide patient with prn assistance to the bathroom.

Proprioception: A non-visual sensation that enables an individual to perceive movement of parts of the body as well as the position of some of the body parts in relation to others.

Proprioceptive neuromuscular facilitation: An exercise incorporating the simultaneous use of a combination of limb activities to help improve neuromuscular function. Typically the exercise involves the use of both strong and weak muscles with the goal of improving strength in the weaker muscles.

Proximal: Structures of the body closest to the brain and spinal cord.

Psychiatrist: A doctor of medicine or osteopathy who specializes in the diagnosis and treatment of behavioral abnormalities and mental diseases. As physicians, psychiatrists can prescribe medication.

Psychologist: A health professional who is trained to diagnose and treat psychological, behavioral, emotional, and social issues. Their areas of practice include psychological testing, educational guidance, and counseling. Psychologists do not prescribe medication.

Ptosis: Drooping of one or both eyelids.

Pulmonary embolism: Passage of blood clots from the veins to the lungs.

Pulmonary function tests: A group of tests used to evaluate breathing function and oxygen delivery to the blood stream.

Pulmonologist: A doctor of medicine or osteopathy who specializes in disorders of the lungs and breathing problems.

Pulse oximeter: A device that measures the amount of oxygen in the blood and helps determine if the patient is receiving enough oxygen. It is a non-invasive test that is very easy to use.

Pulsed treatment: Treatment given intermittently in large doses.

Pyridoxine: Vitamin B^6.

Quadriceps: The large group of muscles on the front of the thigh.

Radicles: *See* nerve roots.

Radiculoneuropathy: A neuropathy that affects the nerve roots as they emerge from the spinal cord as well as the peripheral nerves as they extend further into the limbs.

Radiculopathy: Any abnormality of the nerve roots or radicles.

Range of motion exercise: An exercise in which a joint moves through its maximal amount or range of movement. The exercise can be passive, for the very weak patient, wherein the therapist moves the leg through its range of motion, or the exercise can be active, for the stronger patient, who performs the movement alone or with the assistance of a therapist.

Rehabilitation: Restoration to normal or improved function. In GBS this refers to restoration of physical function.

Rehabilitation medicine: The branch of medicine that deals with the diagnosis and treatment of disease and injury by means of physical agents, such as manipulation, massage, exercise, heat, or water. Often, rehabilitation medicine is also called physical medicine and rehabilitation or physiatry. The physician who specializes in this field is called a physiatrist.

Respiratory rate: The number of breathes that a person takes each minute.

Sacral: Pertaining to the sacrum, the area around the hips and buttocks.

Schwann cell: The cell that produces the myelin sheath in peripheral nerves which is named for the scientist who first identified it.

Segmental: Involving a segment.

Sensory: Pertaining to sensation or feeling.

Septicemia: Infection of the blood.

Skilled nursing facility: A patient care facility that is able to provide a skilled level of nursing and other care. This usually includes some rehabilitation. For GBS patients, this option of care is typically offered when they are too weak to return home, but not strong enough to receive the intensive level of therapy that an acute rehabilitation hospital provides.

Social worker: An individual trained to address the societal interactive issues that typically confront people who are ill or otherwise disabled. In the medical domain, the social worker may play many roles such as analyzing a patient's insurance coverage, identifying medical facilities to provide optimal care, determining a family's ability to handle medical needs at home and providing counseling to patients and families in dealing with medical and social issues. Some social workers are also licensed to perform formal psycho-social counseling.

Spasticity: Stiffness of the muscles caused by damage to the nerves in the central nervous system that control muscle activity.

Speech therapist: A medical professional who is trained to work with patients in restoring speech and communication functions. They also evaluate swallowing disorders and guide patient care relevant to safe and optimal food consistencies.

Speech therapy: A form of therapy that assists patients to restore speech and communication functions.

Spinal tap *See* lumbar puncture.

Stenosis: Narrowing of a tube.

Substitution: The phenomenon whereby stronger muscles are used to compensate for weaker muscles. For example, if hip flexors, the muscles that raise the thigh up and forward, are weak and limit normal walking, a patient can compensate by swinging the leg outwards and pitching forward, using other hip and back muscles to create forward motion. To switch the patient from substitution to normal function, the abnormal motion should be recognized and steps taken to correct it with the use of exercises to strengthen weak muscles.

Supportive care: Treatments given to prevent, control, or relieve problems caused by an illness, its complications and side effects and to improve the patient's comfort and quality of life. Supportive care can be contrasted with disease-specific care, care that is designed to deal with a specific disorder.

Sympathetic nervous system: The part of the autonomic nervous system that controls the body's functions that result from excitement, anger, or fear.

Syncope: Fainting.

Systemic lupus erythematosis (lupus): A rare autoimmune disease that causes arthritis, kidney failure, and skin rashes as well as damage to many other organs, including peripheral nerves.

Systolic blood pressure: The pressure in the arteries recorded during contraction of the heart muscle. The top number of the two numbers recorded when the blood pressure is measured.

Tachycardia: Abnormally rapid heart rate, usually greater than 100 beats per minute.

Testosterone: The major male sex hormone made by the testis or testicles. Testosterone is required to facilitate a normal erection and libido or sex drive. The blood level of testosterone will be decreased if the testicles do not make a sufficient amount or with impaired production of luteinizing hormone, from the pituitary gland at the base of the brain, that drives production of testosterone.

Thrombi: Plural of thrombus.

Thrombosis: Clotting of the blood within the blood vessels.

Thrombus: A blood clot within a blood vessel. In GBS, blood clots usually form within veins and may break off and travel to the lungs causing pulmonary embolism.

Thyroid stimulating hormone: A hormone produced in the pituitary gland that stimulates the thyroid gland to produce thyroid hormones.

Tick paralysis: A rare condition in which severe muscle weakness results from a toxin contained in the saliva of a wood tick.

Tidal volume: The amount of air inhaled or exhaled by a patient with a single normal breath. It is measured in *liters* (1 liter equals approximately 1 quart).

Trachea: The tube that carries air from the nose to the lungs.

Tracheostomy: A surgical procedure on the neck to facilitate safe, long term mechanical ventilation. In a tracheostomy a small cut is made at the base of the neck; a tube is then inserted directly through the skin at this incision into the upper part of the airway or trachea.

Transverse myelitis: A condition in which inflammation of the spinal cord causes weakness and sensory symptoms in those parts of the body below the site of the inflammation.

Tricyclic antidepressants: A class of drugs with a specific chemical structure that is used to treat depression.

T-tube: A T-shaped tube placed over the tracheostomy during the weaning process to provide a high concentration of oxygen in the inspired air.

Tumescence: Swelling. In the context of penile function, swelling of the penis, or its tumescence, along with penile rigidity contribute to an effective erection that enables successful coitus or intercourse.

Ulnar: Pertaining to the ulna bone on the inside of the arm below the elbow.

Ultrasound imaging: A type of imaging that uses ultrasound waves to create pictures of internal organs.

Vasculitis: Inflammation of the blood vessels.

Ventilator: A medical device that supplies artificial breathing. It is attached to the patient via a plastic tube that is inserted into the airway, an endotracheal tube or tracheostomy tube.

Video swallow study: A video x-ray taken during the act of swallowing.

Vital capacity: A measure of breathing function. Often measured as the forced vital capacity (FVC), it is the largest amount of air that can be forced out of the lungs with a strong exhalation following full inspiration. To measure the FVC, the lips are placed firmly on a mouthpiece and the patient exhales as hard as possible.

Vital signs: A group of measurements that provide an index of essential body functions. These measurements are heart (pulse) rate, blood pressure, temperature, and respiratory rate. When pain is a significant part of a patient's medical condition, it has sometimes been called the "fifth vital sign."

Water therapy: The use of water to provide health benefit. In GBS, water therapy consists of the use of a pool as the place where a weak patient can do an initial trial of walking and exercises. The water provides buoyancy that allows the patient to walk with partial weight bearing.

Weaning: The process of gradually withdrawing a patient from artificial breathing using a mechanical ventilator.

West Nile fever: A condition caused by a viral infection that leads to fever, headache, and rarely, muscle weakness. This condition was first discovered in Africa but has spread to many other areas of the world.

Resources

Since most patients and their families have never heard of Guillain-SBarré syndrome prior to experiencing it, they often seek information about it and other related disorders. This chapter lists sources of information specific to GBS as well as information on resources for individuals with a disability, regardless of the cause.

NATIONAL ORGANIZATIONS RELEVANT TO THE GUILLAIN-BARRÉ SYNDROME PATIENT

GBS/CIDP Foundation International

Holly Building, 1041/2 Forrest Avenue, Narberth, PA 19072
Telephone: 610-667-0131 Fax: 610-667-7036
E-mail: info@gbsfi.com Web site: www.gbsfi.com

The GBS Foundation International was founded in 1976 as a support group for patients with Guillain-Barré syndrome. The name was later changed in 2005 to the "GBS/CIDP Foundation International" to better reflect its contributions to the understanding of both of these disorders. The foundation's foremost goal is to address the needs of GBS and CIDP patients and their families. It is a non-profit volunteer organization with chapters across the

United States and around the world. The foundation provides support groups for patients and their families, written information about the disease, and it sponsors regular meetings in the United States that are typically attended by 300 people. Similar meetings are held in other countries. The foundation also has volunteers who visit affected patients during the acute phase of the disease. When a normally-functioning individual who has had GBS walks into the room of a GBS patient who is still paralyzed and perhaps on a ventilator, the visit can provide a level of comfort and optimism to the patient that no amount of reassurance from the treating physician can provide.

The Peripheral Neuropathy Association, Inc.

P.O. Box 26226, New York, NY 10117-3422
Telephone: 212-692-0662 Web site: www.neuropathy.org

The Peripheral Neuropathy Association (PNA) is a national organization in the United States that assists individuals with all types of neuropathy, not just GBS and CIDP.

Information about neuropathies, including GBS, CIDP, and peripheral neuropathy, can be obtained from the National Institute of Neurological Disorders and Stroke (NINDS), available on the web at: www.ninds.nih.gov.

National Organization for Rare Diseases (NORD)

P. O. Box 1968, Danbury, CT 06813-1968
Telephone: 203-744-0100 Web site: www.rarediseases.org

The NORD web site contains useful information and resources about many rare disorders, including Guillain-Barré syndrome.

Disabled Dealer (magazine)
Telephone: 888-651-0666 Web site: www.disableddealer.com

This magazine addresses disability issues and features advertisements for assistive devices.

Australia, New Zealand, and Tasmania

Several support groups and other patient-based organizations are located in these geographic areas. *See* patient newsletter and web site listings below for contact information.

PATIENT NEWSLETTERS

United States

The Communicator, published by the GBS/CIDP Foundation International, Holly Building, 104 1/2 Forrest Ave, Narberth, PA 19072. Telephone: 610-667-0131; Fax: 610-667-7036; E-mail: info@gbsfi.com Web site: www.gbsfi.com.

Australia

Inflammatory Neuropathy Support Group of Victoria, Australia, contains on-line newsletter articles. 138B Princess St. Kew, Victoria 3101, Australia. Contact: James Gerrand, Telephone: +61-3-9853-6443; Fax: +61-3-9853-4150; E-mail: ingroup@vicnet.net.au; Web site: home.vicnet.net.au/~ingroup/welcome.htm .

New Zealand

Newsletter of the Guillain-Barré Syndrome Support Group Trust of New Zealand. 27 Grenville Street, New Plymouth, New Zealand. National Coordinator: Jenny Murray; Telephone/Fax: (06) 751-1014; Email: Jenny.gbs.nz@clear.net.nz.

United Kingdom

Reaching Out, published by the GBS Support Group of the United Kingdom and Ireland. 3 Dingat View; Llandovery, SA20 OBL. Editor: Alan Young, MBE; Telephone: 01550 720698; Fax: 01550 720030; E-mail: alneyoung@aol.com. GBS Support Group offices: LCC offices, Eastgate, Sleaford, Lincolnshire NG34 7EB; UK; Telephone/Fax: +44 1529 304615; E-mail: admin@gbs.org.uk.

WEB SITES

Several web sites provide useful information for patients with GBS and related conditions. Please be aware that information obtained from the Internet may come from sources with biased, inaccurate, and self-interested motives. The organized support groups in the United States, United Kingdom, New Zealand, and elsewhere try to provide authoritative, objective information. The following web sites contain a wealth of information that may be very helpful.

- GBS Support Group of the UK and Ireland: www.gbs.org.uk
- GBS/CIDP Foundation International: www.gbsfi.com
- GBS Support Group of New Zealand: www.nzordgroups.org.nz/guillainbarre/default.asp
- eMedicine site on GBS and rehabilitation, by Angela Cha-Kim, MD: www.emedicine.com/pmr/topic48.htm
- The Inflammatory Neuropathy Support Group of Victoria Inc., Australia: home.vicnet.net.au/~ingroup/welcome.htm
- GBS Association of New South Wales, Australia: www.gbsnsw.org.au/web/home/tabid/52/default.aspx

INSURANCE ISSUES

Insurance issues for the GBS patient fall into several categories, including health, catastrophic, prescription, home care, and income.

INSURANCE COVERAGE

Structure of Insurance Payments

Insurance policies and coverage can be complicated. The language in policies is often written in terms to satisfy the insurance company's legal department rather than helping the patient understand their coverage and rights. If the company denies payment for some service or product that you think is covered under your insurance plan, contact your company representative for an explanation. If you still feel that the company is not honoring your insurance plan correctly, it may be possible to appeal the decision in writing. Determine the person in the company to whom correspondence should be sent, their exact mailing address, spelling of their name, and title. The company will usually provide instructions to make a formal appeal. Some companies may seem to work in a vacuum by denying access to the important people who make decisions. For example, underwriters, the people who look at a patient's risk and decide how much to charge for insurance, typically will not talk to customers. The patient's insurance agent may need to act as an intermediating agent.

When making contact with your insurance company be sure to record the date of the call, the name of the person you spoke with, and the department with phone number or extension. Insurance companies tend to be big and it is easy to get lost in the shuffle when dealing with them.

Suppliers of wheelchairs, orthotics, and other assistive equipment, which are called *durable medical equipment* (DME) by suppliers, will typically have the patient or their representative sign a document when a product is delivered in order to allow the supplier to bill the patient's insurance. If, however, the supplier can not collect from the insurance company, the signed document may give the supplier the right to bill the patient. Before paying the supplier, you may want to send a written appeal or telephone your insurance company to determine the rationale for their decision.

When submitting a request to insurance companies for reimbursement or payment, providers of medical care (doctors, home care agencies, equipment suppliers, etc.) usually use procedure codes to indicate the service(s) performed, and the corresponding code for the diagnosis that warranted the service. These diagnosis codes are listed in the *International Classification of Diseases, Ninth Revision, Clinical Modification* or *ICD-9-CM Codes.* The codes are based on the World Health Organization's classification of diseases. Sometimes the reason for nonpayment by the insurance company is an incorrect diagnosis code, one that does not readily explain the reason the physician prescribed the equipment or provided a service. If payment was declined, look at the diagnosis code for the equipment (if given). Call the vendor and ask what the code signifies to be sure it is correct. If the diagnosis seems to be correct, check with the insurance company as to reason for nonpayment. For example, a diagnosis of Guillain-Barré syndrome, 357.0, may be correct, but not a sufficient reason for the insurance company to pay for a walker. If, however, the diagnosis is paraparesis, 344.1, paralyzed or weak legs, this language and code may be what the insurance company requires in order to cover the item.

Insurance Coverage and Discharge Planning

Insurance companies may on occasion be inclined to minimize a patient's needs, or they may not have a good understanding of a patient's medical status and needs from the reports supplied. They may sometimes be inclined to push for early discharge of a patient from a rehabilitation hospital to home, or from physical therapy at home. Hospital billing personnel, case managers, utilization nurses, and physicians are experienced in dealing with these insurance issues, and can usually adequately inform the company as to the patient's need for continued care in a rehabilitation center or their readiness for discharge. Sometimes the patient or family may feel that the patient is not ready for discharge. Perhaps the family is overwhelmed by the patient's needs, or even the prospect that the patient may not get better, and may have physical disabilities that could last indefinitely. This is a natural concern. Hopefully, prior to a patient's discharge from one facility to the next, the hospital care/case management team and treating physicians have analyzed the patient's medical status and ambulation capabilities, as well as the level of care available at the receiving facility. This information is useful to determine if the patient can get adequate treatment at the next place, even if this is discharge to home. If the family feels differently they may want to discuss this issue with the attending physician, hospital social worker, discharge planner, and utilization/care manager. The attending physician or hospital representative usually has the option to disagree with the insurance company's determination and appeal their decision by phone. On occasion, there may be a need for the patient or their family representative to talk directly with the insurance company about timing and location of discharge. Hospital personnel are usually very experienced in handling these matters. Remember, insurance coverage can determine what options of care will be available for a patient.

Future Insurability

Once recovered, the former GBS patient is essentially back to baseline with respect to their health and longevity, and there should be no problem purchasing health or life insurance. Of course, it is possible that a naïve insurer or the underwriters, the people who determine insurability, may want to "rate" a former GBS patient, that is, charge more than they normally would for a healthy person. If this occurs, it may be beneficial for the former GBS patient to ask their insurance agent to provide the company's underwriters with a note from their physician to document the client's health status and good prognosis.

Hospital and Doctor Bills

The insurance industry has a rather unique, perhaps even peculiar payment arrangement with most hospitals, doctors, equipment suppliers, and other care providers. Many, even most, insurers will usually pay a predetermined amount to these providers, regardless of the dollar amount of the actual bill. Sometimes these amounts have been negotiated in a contract, as between an HMO and a hospital. To make the situation even more confusing, insurance payments by Medicare, Blue Cross, Blue Shield, and some private insurers to doctors are often based upon the providers' prior charges. Therefore, physicians will usually charge more than they expect to get paid; this higher charge enables them to get a higher payment in future years, to offset inflation. The Diagnostic Related Groups (DRG) system is another example of a payment system peculiar to Medicare. Under this system, Medicare pays a hospital based upon the patient's diagnoses, not upon the care given. The hospital may get the same payment, whether the hospital stay was 2 weeks or 3 weeks. The hospital will usually try to document any and all complications that a patient had in order to get more equitable (bigger) payments. When looking at billing and payment records between a hospital, doctor, or other provider and an insurance company, the patient can often overlook the provider's charges. A closer review of the billing statement will show the actual services/care provided and what was actually paid for those services.

THE VACCINE INJURY COMPENSATION PROGRAM

In recognition of the small risk associated with influenza and other immunizations, the United States Congress, in 1986, created a program to compensate individuals who are injured as the result of vaccination. The "Vaccine Injury Compensation Program (VICP)" is designed to settle vaccine injury claims through a no-fault system of compensation as an alternative to the traditional tort system, in which the patient might seek legal judgment against the vaccine manufacturer. For information about this program contact:

National Vaccine Injury Compensation Program

Parklawn Building, 5600 Fishers Lane, Room 11C-26, Rockville, MD 20857

Telephone 800-338-2382

Web site: www.hrsa.gov/osp/vicp/fact_sheet.htm

The National Vaccine Information Center (NVIC) is a national, non-profit educational organization founded to advocate for reform of mass vaccination programs. Persons who feel that they may have developed GBS or CIDP following vaccination may get more information by contacting:

National Vaccine Information Center

412-E Church Street, Vienna, VA 22180

Telephone: 703-938-3783 Fax: 703-938-5768

Web site: www.nvic.org/Default.htm

ADDITIONAL READING

Personal Accounts of Guillain-Barré Syndrome

Availability of these books may be determined by checking with the GBS/CIDP Foundation International office, 610-667-0131, or the publisher.

Baier S, Zimmeth M. *Bed Number Ten.* Holt, Rinehart, & Winston: New York, 1986.

Baier S, Zimmeth M. *Bed Number Ten.* Good Housekeeping: December 1985.

Borshik D. *It Could Be You.* Write-TYPE: Crewe, Cheshire, UK, 1996.

Heller J, Vogel S. *No Laughing Matter.* G. P. Putnam & Sons: New York, 1986. (Out of print).

Langton BS. *A First Step–Understanding Guillain-Barré Syndrome.* Trafford Publishing: Victoria, BC, 2002.

Langton BS, Ondrich S, Hill, P. *Guillain-Barré Syndrome: 5 Years Later.* Trafford Publishing: Victoria, BC, 2006.

Other Books for Laypersons

Steinberg JS. *Guillain-Barré Syndrome—An Overview for the Layperson.* GBS/CIDP Foundation International: Narberth, 2000.

Rummelsburg H. *Guillain-Barré Syndrome, A Handbook for Caregivers.* Available from the GBS/CIDP Foundation International: Narberth.

Schardt P. *Guillain-Barré Syndrome, Caring for a Child with GBS.* Available from the GBS/CIDP Foundation International: Narberth.

Books for Physicians

Hughes RAC. *Guillain-Barré Syndrome.* Springer-Verlag: London, 1990.

Ropper, AH, Wijdicks EFM, Truax, BT. *Guillain-Barré Syndrome.* F. A. Davis Company: Philadelphia, 1991.

Parry GJ. *Guillain-Barré Syndrome.* Thieme Medical Publishers: New York, 1993.

A

C

D

E

F

G

H

O

P

Q

R

W

X

Y

Z

Books For ALL Kinds of Readers

At ReadHowYouWant we understand that one size does not fit all types of readers. Our innovative, patent pending technology allows us to design new formats to make reading easier and more enjoyable for you. This helps improve your speed of reading and your comprehension. Our EasyRead printed books have been optimized to improve word recognition, ease eye tracking by adjusting word and line spacing as well as minimizing hyphenation. Our EasyRead SuperLarge editions have been developed to make reading easier and more accessible for vision-impaired readers. We offer Braille and DAISY formats of our books and all popular E-Book formats.